D0648196

THE
PARTNERSHIP
DIET
PROGRAM

THE PARTNERSHIP DIET PROGRAM

The Do-It-Together
Pounds-Off Program
That Doesn't Feel
Like a Diet

Kelly D. Brownell, Ph.D.
with Irene Copeland

Rawson, Wade Publishers, Inc.
New York

To my parents, Arnold and Margaret, and to Mary Jo

Library of Congress Cataloging in Publication Data

Brownell, Kelly D
   The partnership diet program.

   Includes index.
   1. Reducing diets.   2. Reducing—Psychological
aspects.   3. Friendship—Psychological aspects.
I. Copeland, Irene, joint author. II. Title.
RM222.2.B785 1979   613.2'5   79-64200
ISBN 0-89256-103-3

Published simultaneously in Canada by McClelland and
   Stewart, Ltd.
Composition by American–Stratford Graphic Services, Inc.
   Brattleboro, Vermont
Printed and bound by Fairfield Graphics,
   Fairfield, Pennsylvania
Designed by Gene Siegel
First Edition

Acknowledgments

I have many people to thank for their contributions to the writing of this book. Their support has made the task gratifying and enjoyable. Judy Billingsley, Beth Venditti, and Janet Albaum are to be congratulated for their patience in collecting information, making telephone calls, and typing portions of the manuscript. Freddy Kaye, M.S., and Dr. Eleanor Whitney provided useful information about nutritional matters. I am grateful for the collaboration of Drs. Carol L. Heckerman, Robert J. Westlake, Steven C. Hayes, and Peter M. Monti for their assistance with the study that gave birth to this book. I welcome this opportunity to pay tribute to my teachers and colleagues, Drs. G. Terence Wilson, Albert J. Stunkard, David H. Barlow, Sandra L. Harris, and Arnold A. Lazarus. They have had a very positive influence on my thinking, research, teaching, and clinical practice. Special thanks are due Dr. G. Terence Wilson whose ideas and intellectual stimulation helped form the very basis of this book. Finally, the most heartfelt appreciation goes to Mary Jo Brownell. Her loving support during my long hours at the typewriter and her kind regard for my personal and professional endeavors have been invaluable.

Foreword

Behavioral methods of weight reduction were introduced just over a decade ago and, in this time, they have revolutionized the approach to weight control. Crash diets and magical formulas still enjoy their brief commercial successes, but they are no more effective in keeping weight off than they ever were. As a result, more and more people are turning to behavioral methods for the slower but more enduring weight losses that they foster.

Over half a million Americans each week take part in commercial weight-reduction programs that use behavioral principles, and many others use behavioral self-help manuals. These developments have made weight loss easier and more lasting for large numbers of people. But they leave much to be desired. Behavioral programs are difficult to learn and there is rarely enough time to learn them. Even the hour or two a week provided by the commercial weight-loss groups is pitifully little to pit against the constant pressures to eat with which we are assaulted daily in our affluent society. And when discouragement and faltering resolve threaten the continuation of a weight-reduction program, there is, all too often, no one who knows how to help.

Dr. Brownell's recognition that adding social support to a behavioral program might increase its effectiveness both in losing weight and in keeping it off was a singularly valuable insight. Here is a way of making it easier to learn the behavioral procedures and to counteract the enormous environmental pressures to overeat. If all goes well, it is a way of developing and strengthening bonds of friendship and love. The Partnership Diet provides the opportunity for sharing experiences that can deepen any relationship.

One of the most important experiences is that of keeping a diet diary. As Dr. Brownell points out, the diet diary is the single most important part of the program—and for a good reason. It makes one aware of things that would otherwise go unnoticed. And the number of things that can go unnoticed, without this special effort, is often sufficient to destroy even the most ardent effort at losing weight. I remember some years ago an overweight woman who had finished a psychoanalysis that had benefited her greatly and that had sharpened her skills at self-examination. But it was only when she kept a diet diary that she realized how much she ate, and when and where and why.

Sharing the learning of the other behavioral techniques should make the task easier and should make the relationship stronger. It is inconvenient and exasperating to put one's fork down between bites, to leave food on one's plate, to shop only in certain specified ways. But it is helpful in losing weight and, as valuable, it gives a sense of mastery, of control over one's life, that is all too rare. Sharing experiences is good for any partnership. Sharing experiences of mastery and self-control is even better. Best of all is the shared experience of losing weight and keeping it off. The Partnership Diet Program provides this opportunity.

Albert Stunkard, M.D.
Professor of Psychiatry
University of Pennsylvania

Contents

ure. You can learn to count calories and eat more deliciously than ever before.

PART 1

The Principles of
Partnership Dieting

CHAPTER 1

The Weight-Loss Program That Really Works

My Partnership Diet Program should be the last weight-reducing system you will ever need. This revolutionary approach is based on one fact—Together Is Better!

Are you skeptical? I don't blame you. Your friends, family, lover, co-workers, etc. (potential partners for the program) are probably skeptical too. They have seen you diet before. By the time I see a patient in private consultation or in one of my clinics, he or she has tried an average of ten different programs and countless "self-help" diets. If any had really worked, my clinics would not have such long waiting lists.

Your experience has probably been similar. I doubt that this is the first diet book you have read. I imagine you have tried many diets before. If you had truly succeeded, you would not be reading this book now.

And for the partners, you have tried many ways to help. In fact, there are psychological adaptations that partners make when dealing with a dieter (more about this later). When the dieter fails to lose weight, the partner can be every bit as frustrated and disappointed as the dieter.

Why have all these diets failed? The answer is simple.

You didn't fail. *The diet failed you.* You did not do anything wrong. The diet was wrong. Your first order of business is to banish the blame that you put on your own shoulders. The Partnership Program will work for you!

3

Any Diet That Restricts Your Eating Is Destined to Fail

It doesn't matter whether you followed your doctor's diet, or one you read about, or simply tried to cut calories on your own. Were you on a no-carbohydrate diet, a high-protein diet, a liquid protein fast, a grapefruit diet, a rice diet, an eight-glasses-of-water-a-day diet? They all have one or more built-in flaws—I call them failure factors—that sabotage your most persistent efforts.

Failure Factor #1. Any restrictive diet that dictates what you must eat and what you must not eat is usually so unappetizing and so boring—and may even be so dangerous —that you simply cannot stay on it long enough to reach your goal.

Failure Factor #2. Restrictive diets don't teach you new eating habits that prepare you for the real world. The result: you start gaining as soon as you stop dieting because you slide right back into the old eating habits that made you gain in the first place.

Failure Factor #3. Even if you follow a sensible, well-balanced diet that allows you to continue eating some of the foods you enjoy, you still don't get what you really need: the emotional support and day-to-day encouragement to keep up the lonely, boring, long-term diet process. This is where the partner comes in.

What happens? You become a yo-yo dieter. See if you recognize some of your patterns in these profiles of two of my patients.

"I know I can lose weight. I've done it dozens of times."

Stephanie was a chubby baby and a plump teen-ager. When she finished college and went to work at an advertising agency, she made an unsettling discovery: an overweight youngster might be cute, but an overweight career woman was just plain heavy and was at a real disadvantage.

Determined to lose weight, Stephanie went from one doctor to another, looking for help. The first simply gave her a follow-up appointment six months away and told her to lose fifty pounds. A second doctor gave her a meal plan, but the meals were so boring she could stay on the diet only a few days at a time and then would binge on her favorite foods. A third doctor gave her a rainbow-hued assortment of pills, but a newspaper article about the dangers of diet pills frightened her into throwing them out.

Stephanie bought diet books and followed each new diet scheme that came along. Each one worked initially when she was optimistic and determined. But after losing ten or twenty pounds, she became bored or discouraged and rebounded quickly to her old weight. She was so distraught by her failures that she had no hope of ever being thin. By the time she entered my program, Stephanie estimated that she had gained and lost more than six hundred pounds in her lifetime.

"If you love me, eat."

Felicia's parents are both overweight, and so is her brother. She had to finish everything on her plate, even if she wasn't hungry. Her mother regarded leftovers as a personal insult.

Felicia learned very early to celebrate happy times with food and to use food for solace during sad times. Despite the fact that she was practically force-fed, she was so active on the swimming team and in other competitive sports during her school years that she managed to keep her weight under control.

Her 125-pound shape expanded rapidly when she married Joe. Felicia thought being a good wife meant serving Joe elaborate dinners every night, topped off with special desserts she baked herself. She ate right along with him, in addition to snacking during the day. Although she tried to continue her swimming, without the incentive of competition, and with a baby to care for, she became less and less active.

Felicia hated her body, but every time she started a diet

and managed to lose a few pounds, something would happen to set her back. Joe would bring home a big box of candy and she would polish it off to avoid hurting him. When her mother-in-law invited them to dinner, Felicia felt she had to eat as much as everyone else.

Yo-Yo Dieting Is Dangerous to Your Health

Throughout my years of research into the treatment of obesity, supervising weight-reduction groups, and doing intensive therapy with individuals, I have been discouraged by this yo-yo phenomenon. My colleagues, and of course my patients, shared my disappointment.

Many people feel that if they lose twenty pounds and then gain it back they are no worse off than before. You may feel the same. Not true! Although more research is needed on this subject, you may do more damage to your body by losing weight and gaining it back than by simply staying overweight—especially when you repeat the process.

When I realized how little attention had been paid to the possible harmful effects of yo-yo dieting, I decided to make a special study of the medical and psychological implications of the pounds-off, pounds-on syndrome. Here are the sobering facts:

During periods of weight gain, blood pressure and serum cholesterol show substantial increases. Both are major risk factors for coronary heart disease. Experiments with laboratory animals have shown that serious heart problems can be associated with repeated episodes of dramatic weight loss followed by rapid weight gain. These problems include electrocardiogram abnormalities, erratic heart rate and blood pressure, and chronic hypertension. In a more extreme example, humans who have gone through periods of enforced starvation suffer high rates of heart disease during the "refeeding" period.

The implication is clear; the cumulative effect of many episodes of weight loss followed by weight gain may result in damage to the cardiovascular system. The problems may develop during periods of weight gain, the time when you are least likely to have medical supervision.

There is another compelling reason to avoid yo-yo dieting. When you lose weight rapidly, especially when you diet without exercising, you lose lean body tissue (muscle) as well as fat, because your body cannot mobilize your stored-up fat fast enough. When you regain weight your body can produce fat more quickly than lean tissue, so much of the excess energy (calories) is converted to fat. With each rebound a greater percentage of your body becomes fat. I have found that few of my patients relish this muscle-to-blubber image.

Yo-yo dieting can create psychological problems as well. Just being on a diet is emotionally stressful. In various controlled studies dieters have reported feelings of nervousness, depression, anxiety, irritability, anger, frustration, and preoccupation with food. It is understandable that an ineffective diet can cause even more distress.

Here is a situation I see very often: a patient loses weight on a diet and attributes the weight loss, not to his or her own efforts, but to the magical properties of the diet. Partners tend to feel the same way. When weight is regained, it is not the diet that is blamed, but the dieter's own lack of "will power." This adds still another "failure experience" to a history of aborted diet attempts. No wonder yo-yo dieters feel discouraged, depressed, guilty, ineffectual, and angry. It's no wonder partners feel frustrated.

In working with overweight patients, I have always been troubled by their suffering. They try so hard, and conventional treatments just don't work. Fortunately I have been in a position to conduct research and run test programs until I could find a way to eliminate the failure factors of existing weight-loss systems and help dieters escape the yo-yo trap. The result is the Partnership Diet Program which I am sharing with you in this book.

How the Partnership Diet Program Was Developed

The breakthrough came in 1975 at Brown University in Rhode Island. With two colleagues, I set up a weight-reduction clinic that produced surprising and remarkable results.

During my previous work with overweight people at Rutgers University, I had experimented with behavior modification techniques and had been frustrated by the inconsistency of the results.

You probably have heard about behavioral diet programs—perhaps even been involved in one. The basic approach is to teach new eating habits, or behaviors, to replace the old ones that caused the excess weight. Briefly (you will read much more about this later), *what* you eat is important. But *how* (slowly instead of at Olympic speed), *when* (at planned mealtimes instead of any old time), and *where* (at the dining table instead of in front of the TV set) are also crucial factors.

Scientists generally agree that behavior modification techniques hold the most promise for overweight people. It is the best approach we know of so far . . . but a program can be best and still not work as well as it should. I was determined to improve on the basic behavioral approach.

Looking back on my experience with dieters, it seemed that many of the best "losers" had something in common. Here are two success stories that clued me in.

Nancy had tried at least twenty diets, but the time I first saw her she weighed 185 pounds (on a 5'5" frame). I used the standard behavioral procedures with her for nearly three months, and although she found the new eating behaviors quite helpful, her interest would start to fade every week or two, and so would her ability to stick with the program.

Finally Nancy's husband, Russ, decided to take an active role. He knew his wife wanted to look fabulous at their daughter's wedding, eight months away. So Russ stopped snacking in front of Nancy, went food shopping with her to steer her away from the cookies, kept track of how well she was following the program, and took her to a movie every time she had a particularly good week. He even asked to attend Nancy's sessions so he could learn how to be more supportive.

As soon as Russ became closely involved, there was a dramatic change; Nancy started to lose weight steadily. She weighed 130 pounds at her daughter's wedding.

Two other patients, Susie and Joyce, became friends after meeting in a group I was conducting. By the eighth week of the ten-week program, Susie had lost six pounds and Joyce eight. Both were unhappy because they wanted to lose faster.

As an experiment, I suggested that they team up and use a buddy system to help each other follow the program. They would talk every night on the phone and compare notes on the day's eating, plan the next day's meals, and give each other tips for coping with potential problems like a business trip or a cocktail party.

I kept in touch with these two for several months after our official program ended. Susie eventually lost thirty-two pounds and Joyce twenty-eight.

Nancy, Susie, and Joyce learned *how* to eat from the behavioral program. I realized, however, that the social support each received from a partner gave them the additional motivation to stay with the program.

At the same time that I was observing this phenomenon, other researchers were suggesting that social support could be a useful tool for dieters. But nobody had tested this approach.

With Dr. G. Terence Wilson of Rutgers University, I completed the first controlled study of Partnership Dieting.

In our program each dieter brought the same family member to each of our eight weekly meetings.

We were extremely optimistic . . . but disappointed at the results. Our dieters did no better than a comparison group where dieters attended meetings alone.

We finally isolated the problem: the family members clearly wanted to help, but we had not provided them with specific instructions for partnering. Did being supportive mean buying the dieter a hot fudge sundae when the craving set in, or devising an activity that would distract the dieter's attention from food? Was the partner supposed to ask for an accounting of the day's calories, or wait for the information to be volunteered?

When I arrived at Brown University, I felt I knew how to remedy the problem. This would finally be *the* program to help dieters get rid of their unwanted pounds.

As before, dieters and spouses were trained in behavioral techniques, but this time they were given specific guidelines for working together. Partners received a lengthy manual that described in detail all the ways they could help the dieter.

Result? The dieters in the special partners group lost significantly more weight than dieters who attended similar meetings without a partner. In fact, weight losses for the partnership dieters were nearly *triple* those reported in previous controlled studies. Even more important, a two-year follow-up of these dieters showed that they maintained their weight losses well, demonstrating that the Partnership Diet Program was the most successful for long-term weight change.

Since joining the faculty at the University of Pennsylvania, I have continued this work, and recent research has confirmed the earlier results.

What does this mean for you?

Behavior modification techniques can be useful for many dieters—but not all. The buddy system alone can be useful for some people—but not all. By combining these two powerful approaches, I believe I have created a system that can make the frustrations—and dangers—of weight gain only a bad memory.

What This Book Will Do for You

This book is a step-by-step guide to your own personalized Partnership Diet Program.

You will learn how to select the most supportive partner, and how to help your partner help you succeed. The partner will learn specific methods for aiding in the effort.

You will take my special seven-day course in proven weight-loss techniques designed to help you eat, think, and act like a thin person, so you can stay at your desired weight for a lifetime.

You and your partner will learn my crisis control techniques, troubleshooting tactics for dealing with crises that threaten to destroy your diet. *You* can become the master of your own eating life.

And you will learn—through specialized calorie charts, menus, and recipes—just how *sumptuously* you can eat.

I know the Partnership Diet Program can work for you, just as it has worked for so many others.

Some of My Favorite Success Stories

Couple Loses Ninety-two Pounds in Twenty-four Weeks

Sally, a chronic nibbler, was depressed about being overweight. She had tried everything from hypnosis to a liquid protein diet, but nothing ever worked.

"After losing five pounds I wanted everybody to tell me how great I looked. But five pounds never showed. The rewards for dieting didn't make up for the suffering, so I never stuck it out."

Martin, Sally's boyfriend, never had a weight problem until a serious accident at work kept him inactive for several months. The new experience of being fat not only made him miserable but it gave him firsthand insight into the problems Sally had been having, and into the importance of praise and encouragement.

Martin insisted that the two of them join one of my Partnership Diet groups. In twenty-four weeks, Sally lost forty-two pounds and Martin lost fifty. Two months later when they came back for a checkup, Sally had lost an additional five pounds and Martin had maintained his weight to the pound.

Sally reported the hardest part of the program was trying to explain it to people who asked, "What did you have to give up?" "They thought I was kidding when I said 'nothing,' but it's really true. And with Martin telling me every day how neat I was looking, and what terrific meals I was cooking, I really can't say I suffered."

Reluctant Partner Loses Twenty-nine Pounds

Harry was a paunchy 210 pounds when he agreed to come to a partners group "to help Milly lose those twenty pounds she's always moaning about."

At 6'1", Harry didn't really think he was fat, just cuddly. "Heck, I'm a salesman," he told the group. "People expect a salesman to be jolly and a little round."

Milly worried constantly that his long hours of traveling and the crazy meals he ate on the road were making him a candidate for a heart attack. But she didn't want to nag.

After a few weeks of helping Milly lose weight, Harry found that just by not snacking in front of Milly, and by making other efforts to help her, he had lost nine pounds. He sheepishly admitted that he felt better and was going to follow the program himself. At the end of ten weeks, he was down to a trim 181 pounds.

The Partnership Diet Program Helps a Marriage

Judy hated leaving Houston when her husband's company transferred him to Philadelphia. She found a job in a day-care center but she was lonely without her friends and family, and Irwin often worked late. Out of boredom, she would start to snack as soon as she got home at four o'clock. On the nights Irwin worked late she made dinner for herself, then made something for him when he got home and nibbled while he ate.

Irwin was upset because Judy was losing her slim figure. He kept telling her, "Why don't you just eat less!" He didn't mean to be cruel, but he couldn't understand her lack of "will power." Because he didn't know how to cope with Judy's problem, he found excuses to work late even more often. Finally, after a number of serious arguments, and after Judy had gained sixty pounds, they went to a marriage counselor.

At the same time a neighbor encouraged the couple to join one of my groups. Irwin was reluctant at first. "It's not my fault she's fat," he insisted. But after some persuasion by Judy and the marriage counselor, he signed up.

As soon as Irwin heard the stories of other dieters in the group, he realized that Judy was no "weaker" than anyone else. He also saw that by avoiding the problem he was only making it worse.

Once Irwin's attitude began to change, Judy began losing weight. He still works late occasionally, but when he does he calls to chat. More often he brings work home so he can be with her. Judy is working on a master's degree and now the two do their homework together.

Both claim their marriage is much happier, partly because of the marriage counseling and partly because of their joint efforts to help Judy lose weight. Her thirty-seven-pound loss in sixteen weeks is an accomplishment they are both proud of—and they both are still working toward her sixty-pound goal.

The Rest of Stephanie's Story

Under my supervision, Stephanie (the yo-yo dieter I told you about earlier) learned how to get help from two important partners. One was her roommate, Rhoda, and the other a co-worker, Helen.

Rhoda monitored the refrigerator to keep tempting snacks out of sight, and she gave Stephanie backgammon lessons to take her mind off snacking.

Helen kept Stephanie away from the coffee wagon at the office by filling her cup for her, and searched out nearby restaurants with sensible menus where they could lunch together.

It took a year, but Stephanie has lost fifty-four pounds —and discovered what really good friends she has.

The Rest of Felicia's Story

Felicia, the yo-yo dieter who didn't want to hurt anyone by refusing to eat, had to learn to think of herself. She asked Joe to show his affection by bringing flowers home instead of candy, and even more important, by helping her when she needed support.

Joe practices all of the new eating behaviors with Felicia. He told both sets of in-laws that he and Felicia would feel just as loved and pampered when they came to visit if the meals were less lavish. He also tries to keep Felicia out of the kitchen as much as possible.

Felicia is down to 126 pounds, teaches swimming two nights a week at the local Y, and no longer thinks "food is love."

Why the Partnership Diet Program Works

There are three primary reasons for the outstanding success record of Partnership Dieting.

1. *There Are No No-Nos*

My patients complain of diets with an "eat anything on this list" list, or a list of forbidden foods that happens to include all their favorite ingestibles. The foods I have listed here are forbidden on many weight-loss regimens, but with Partnership Dieting you do not have to forsake them:

Butter, margarine,
    cooking oil, shortening
Cakes and pies
Candy
Chocolate
Cookies
Ice cream, sherbet, frozen
    custard
Jellies and jams

Mayonnaise and salad
    dressings
Peanut butter
Pasta (spaghetti,
    macaroni, noodles)
Potatoes (white, sweet,
    yams)
Rice

Go ahead, eat that slice of pizza or that piece of layer cake. With Partnership Dieting you have no reason to feel deprived if you don't—or guilty if you do.

I can hear you saying, "Okay, what's the catch?" The catch is that you eat these high-calorie or high-carbohydrate foods in moderation, within your daily calorie allotment. (You will read more about that in Chapter 4.) But since they are not *forbidden,* you will find that you won't crave them desperately.

Knowing you can eat them, you are more likely to eat them in moderation, and when you do eat them, it doesn't mean that you have fallen off your diet. This approach gives you and your partner the most flexibility.

2. *You Learn New Habits that Help*
   You Enjoy LESS Food MORE

As I have indicated, well-controlled research with dieters has shown that behavioral programs are better than other programs. I have incorporated the best of the behavioral techniques—specifically tailored for Partnership Dieters—in this program, and have designed *new habit-changing behaviors as well.* Our goal is a new eating lifestyle that will help you live comfortably and will help create a pounds-off atmosphere between you and your partner.

Here is an example of how—and why—this habit changing works:

Have you been a fast eater all your life? Many overweight people habitually clean their plates faster than anyone else at the table. You can unlearn this bad habit and learn a new one—eating more slowly. Eating slowly will allow you really to taste your food and enjoy it more. Almost without realizing it, you will be eating less than before.

Your eating speed is an important factor . . . and so are many other aspects of your food-related life, including what you do while you prepare and eat food, how you handle eating urges, how much energy you expend each day, and how you feel when you stick with a diet (and when you don't). In fact, these are so crucial that I have devoted an entire chapter to each one and to others that I use in my clinics.

Finally, this program goes far beyond ordinary behavioral programs because of the most powerful anti-failure factor of all: the Partnership Diet concept.

3. *With Partnership Dieting the Loneliness of the Long-Distance Dieter Is Over*

It is so difficult to stay with a diet because the rewards are very remote. Deny yourself the fattening foods you love and you can look forward to a figure your friends will envy, better health, and perhaps even a longer life. But all of these wonderful benefits are off in the distance. Eat something you crave and the payoff is immediate.

How do you get a reward *now* for slimmanship? That is what the Partnership Diet Program is all about.

I will give you new habits that can reshape your figure and restructure your eating lifestyle. I will show you how to teach the people you love to please you, and how to help them help you to lose weight.

Every time you learn a new slimming behavior, you will learn how to get your partner's help in practicing it. I will show you how to elicit the loving support you need to help you stick with your diet: the compliments, affection, encouragement when you're down, and cheers when you're up.

Many of my patients have been amazed at the subtle changes in their intimate relationships, especially the increased closeness that comes from asking a loved one for help and from working together toward a goal.

Shared experiences are a potent force for bringing people closer and for enriching the quality of a relationship. Now, perhaps for the first time in your life, you will learn how to get someone totally on your side, so that losing weight is no longer a lonely, torturous process, but an enthusiastically shared experience.

I am convinced that my Partnership Diet Program offers you the best chance of slimming without suffering and staying slim without pain.

CHAPTER 2

How to Form a Diet Partnership

This book is based on research and many hours with my patients. Through the struggles of my patients I have learned that the Partnership Diet Program offers you the best chance to change your eating lifestyle and to learn to control your weight.

If you have a mate—are married to or living with someone—or a roommate, that person is the most logical one to be your partner. The two of you share many meals and much of your time, so a live-in partner is most likely to be around when you are confronted with food and when you need encouragement and support. This is the person whose approval may mean the most to you, so you will tend to work extra hard to achieve it. You can expect that the person who cares most about you will make a special effort to help you accomplish something that means so much to you.

What if you live alone or with your family? You can form diet program partnerships with many of the significant people in your life; and later in this chapter I will show you how.

How can you tell ahead of time who the best partner will be? To help you decide, I have developed two special questionnaires for mate and nonmate partnerships. You will find both in this chapter.

18

Can the Partnership Diet Program Improve Your Mate Relationship?

There are two good reasons why it should. One reason, of course, is the experience of sharing. Sharing such an important program can bring you even closer to someone you love. You both can take pride in accomplishing your goals.

The other reason: many overweight people are depressed about their failure to lose. These feelings can make life more difficult for the partners as well as the dieters.

One of my most interesting patients, Rene, said, "I became so irritable when I'd diet that my old boyfriend would have to leave the house. I thought it was him, but now that I am living with Don, the same thing happened until I tried the Partnership Diet."

Once you are confident that you can shed those excess pounds, a relationship can become more relaxed and happy.

Here are two examples of good relationships that became even better after the couples joined my Partnership Diet Program and found new interests to share.

Beth and Steve knew they were watching too much television and not making the most of their evenings—they were in a rut. They were concerned about their expanding waistlines, caused by their habit of snacking while watching TV.

After starting their Partnership Diet, Beth and Steve realized that cutting down on TV time and increasing their activity would help them reach their weight goals more quickly. They made a pact to watch no more than one hour of TV each night, with an additional hour once or twice a week for something special. To use up more calories, they took a nightly walk. This led to an interest in jogging when they discovered that the park near their home had a cinder track for runners.

The result: last Christmas Beth and Steve gave each other matching warm-up suits. They are working on increasing their endurance and plan to run in a six-mile race next year. They are both slimmer now and are much more energetic and involved in a variety of community activities. Recently Steve told me that they have so much to talk about these days that they hardly watch TV at all.

Marie had only one complaint about her otherwise harmonious marriage: Arnie always sat in the living room reading the evening paper while she prepared dinner in the kitchen.

Once they became Partnership Dieters, Arnie realized that he could help Marie lose weight by reducing her involvement with food.

As a bachelor, Arnie had enjoyed cooking for himself, but since marrying Marie—a great cook—he had stayed out of the kitchen. He decided to brush up his cooking skills, and now he prepares the main dish nearly every evening, while Marie cooks the rest of the meal.

They enjoy the challenge of cutting calories in their favorite recipes. (See Chapter 16 for my low-calorie recipes.) With Arnie keeping her company in the kitchen, Marie is less likely to nibble while she cooks.

Most mates make loving and supportive diet partners, whether they have excess pounds of their own to lose or not. Some may not be able to provide the necessary understanding and support. (You will read about one example later.) This quiz, based in part on relationship compatibility questionnaires, will give you some clues as to how hard you will have to work to make your partnership a success. Take the quiz and I will explain your score.

MATE PARTNERSHIP QUIZ

(check one answer for each question)

1) When I am trying to diet and we are around fattening foods, my mate

_____ A. Congratulates me when I show restraint.

3

_____ B. Makes no comment.
2

_____ C. Asks me to try some because "it won't
1   hurt."

2) When I say I am going to start a diet, my mate might say,

_____ A. Terrific, it will make you feel better.
3

_____ B. I hope it works.
2

_____ C. What's the use, I've heard it all before.
1

3) When I complain about being fat, my mate is most likely to say,

_____ A. Why don't we do something to help you
3   with the problem.

_____ B. You're not fat. You look OK to me.
2

_____ C. You're always complaining, but you're still
1   fat.

4) When I am dieting, my mate is most likely to bring home

_____ A. Flowers.
3

_____ B. Nothing.
2

_____ C. Something very sweet and fattening.
1

5) When we are around other people and the subject of dieting and weight comes up, my mate

_____ A. Changes the subject or says something nice
3   about me.

_____ B. Talks about other dieters.
2

_____ C. Tells people my weight problem is hopeless.
1

Check How Often You and Your Mate
Agree on These Issues

(check only one answer for each question)

	Always Agree	Sometimes Agree	Never Agree
6) Money	3	2	1
7) Friends and Social Life	3	2	1
8) Sex	3	2	1
9) Demonstrations of Affection	3	2	1
10) Relatives	3	2	1

11) How happy are you with your relationship?

Extremely Happy 13	Moderately Happy 10	Neither Happy nor Unhappy (7)	Moderately Unhappy 4	Extremely Unhappy 1

12) If you had it to do over, would you become involved with the same person?

Definitely 10	Maybe 5	Absolutely Not 1

How to Score the Mate Partnership Quiz

There is a number below the answers for each question. For example, in questions 1 through 5, each A response is worth 3 points, each B response is worth 2 points, and each C response is worth 1 point. Determine your final score by adding the points for your responses to all twelve questions. (Be sure to total your answers to all the questions.)

Compare your total score to these ranges, then read the explanations that follow.

Score	Conclusion
45 to 53	Your mate is an extremely good choice for the Partnership Program.
32 to 44	Your mate is a good candidate for the Program.
20 to 31	Your mate is a questionable partner for the Program.
12 to 19	Your mate is a doubtful partner for the Program.

If you scored between 45 and 53, your relationship is on very solid ground and your mate will probably be a loving and supportive diet partner.

If you scored between 32 and 44—a reasonably high score—your mate may be a helpful partner. If you scored the fewest points on the first five questions—those involving areas that relate directly to dieting—discuss these questions with your mate and decide jointly whether you should proceed.

If you scored between 20 and 31, your mate is a questionable partner and you should proceed with caution. A score in this range indicates that your mate may be less than helpful in diet-related situations, or that you disagree on other important matters. Your mate *may* turn out to be a valuable partner; before deciding, ask him or her to look through this book to see what the program involves.

If you scored between 12 and 19, there are enough serious disagreements to make a cooperative venture very difficult. You should eliminate your mate as a diet partnership candidate and choose a friend instead. Only in very rare instances should a mate be chosen as a partner if you score below 20. Remember that the Partnership Diet Program requires commitment and effort from both halves of the team, not just from the dieter.

Improving Partner Relations

Some partnerships start off rockily but end up working smoothly. That was the case with Dorothy and Tom.

Dorothy weighed 160 pounds on her wedding day, and for the next twenty-two years she never wavered more than five pounds in either direction. But when their two children went off to college, she decided the time had come to slim down. At the same time she signed up for a secretarial refresher course at the local high school.

Tom had always been a thoughtful and loving husband. Suddenly he became irritable and demanding, and even insisted that Dorothy cook elaborate meals for his parents every weekend. He came home nearly every night with cake or a box of cookies, and he placed bowls of candy and nuts around the living room and den, "in case somebody stops by."

When Dorothy spoke about wanting to lose weight, Tom cut her off with a compliment ("You look just fine to me. You've hardly changed since we got married.") or a discouraging remark ("You like food too much to stay on a diet.").

Dorothy kept calm because she understood what was bothering her husband. Now that both children were out of the house, she and Tom were more dependent on each other. She was trying to improve her figure and was planning to go back to work. Tom's desire to maintain the status quo was not surprising—one more major change (her weight) might be very unsettling.

With great tact and patience, Dorothy managed to reassure her husband that she would still be the same loving wife—and probably a happier and healthier one—if she was thinner. Finally, with Tom's support, she managed to lose twenty-eight pounds.

Few men deliberately try to keep their mates fat. But hidden fears like the ones below can cause a mate to undermine a weight-loss effort even without realizing it.

Will a newly trim and attractive partner suddenly become appealing to the opposite sex?

Will he or she make more physical and emotional demands?

Will a successful dieter make new friends and have a social life that excludes the partner?

Will a trimmer mate become more competitive and independent?

Changes can be upsetting to anyone, but if your potential partner seems overly threatened by your desire to slim down, take these positive steps:

1. Tell your partner the reasons you want to lose weight: your desire to exert some control over what you eat and not be at the mercy of food, your wish to look better in your clothes, and the need to feel more energetic.

2. Remind your partner that excess weight can endanger your health, even shorten your life.

3. Reassure your partner by continuing to display unabated love and affection.

4. Avoid implying that your mate is responsible for your weight problem.

Although any person who is close to you can unwittingly contribute to a weight gain or sabotage a diet effort, remember that ultimately *you* are responsible for your own eating habits. You must make the *major* effort to change.

Nonmate Diet Partnerships

Even if you don't happen to be one half of a couple—or if you decide that your other half won't make a helpful partner—there is no need to travel down life's diet highway alone! Your life is probably crowded with women friends, men friends, relatives, co-workers, neighbors who can be partners.

Before involving yourself in a partnership situation, ask yourself these three questions about any potential partner:

1. Is this person available to me?

Can you call for help day or night, during the week or on weekends? A potential partner should be able to commit both time and emotional involvement to your effort.

Don't rely too heavily on someone who is extremely busy. A friend who is studying for the bar exam or struggling to finish a novel may want to help—but simply may not have the time to be there when you need support.

Avoid choosing friends who are preoccupied with important matters of their own. There will be times when you will need help, and these people can be eager for center stage themselves.

2. Is this person interested in losing weight?

The Partnership Diet Program works whether one or both partners are dieting. But if the two of you are following the program, your motivation and involvement may be even stronger; and each of you may profit from the experience.

However, be cautious in your approach to an overweight friend. He or she may feel you are making a critical comment about his or her weight if you suggest dieting together. And an overweight partner who is not actively participating may unconsciously try to undermine your efforts just to keep you in the same boat.

A slim friend may be a very understanding and helpful partner. But some thin people, particularly those who have never been heavy, may not understand how difficult it is to lose weight. You may hear comments like, "It's easy to lose weight. Just don't eat so much." Be patient: some skinny people are very receptive to training!

3. Is this person really on my side?

When Gail was deciding which friend to ask for help, she quickly eliminated some of the people closest to her. "Iris is a good friend but so terribly self-disciplined; she has no patience with people who are the least bit disorganized. She would be too critical of any setback. I can't ask my sister, Ruth, either. Even though we're devoted to each other, there's a little jealousy there. I'm the youngest, and she thinks our parents favored me."

Gail's ultimate choice was a co-worker she had known only a year. "The fact that we work together so closely makes us great friends. I had a feeling she would be really tuned in to my wanting to lose weight, and I was right. She's been absolutely wonderful."

To help *you* select the most helpful partner, I have developed a questionnaire that will tell you who your real friends are! But first, consider all the partnership possibilities:

Parents As Partners

Parents can be warm and supportive partners—if they are warm and supportive parents. But if they taught you your bad eating habits in the first place, they may not be ready to change. Their lack of sympathy may be discouraging. Some of my patients say their parents (particularly mothers) are the harshest critics.

If you live at home, you may have to shop for your own groceries and cook your own meals in order to avoid the heavy meals coming out of your mother's kitchen.

If you live away from home, you are on your own in the kitchen. Be prepared for possible scare tactics during your visits home. If you turn down a high-calorie food, you may hear this: "You'll get sick if you don't eat right. Why are you starving yourself? You never eat what I make for you."

Children As Partners

A change in the status quo can be difficult for youngsters, especially teen-agers. A fat, comfortable parent who suddenly seems bent on losing weight is definitely a change. Make sure you explain exactly why you want to lose weight. Tell your children they can help by getting their own snacks and by keeping food out of your way as much as possible. A small child following you around with a Twinkie in each hand is not much help, but a responsible child who gets caught up in your weight-loss effort *can* be.

Be especially supportive of an overweight youngster who wants to serve as your partner and to lose weight with you. If sensible eating habits can be formed early, your child is more likely to be free of weight problems later in life.

Other Relatives As Partners

You know the old saying: "You can pick your friends but your relatives are wished on you." Any relative who is on your side can be a helpful partner—if the relative is a friend.

One of my star patients formed an extremely productive partnership with, of all people, her mother-in-law. Sympathetic phone calls and low-cal lunches with this warm, supportive woman helped her lose forty-two pounds in five months.

Roommates As Partners

You may spend as much time with a roommate as you would with a marriage mate. After all, you live together and share meals, a refrigerator, and a pantry. A good roommate-partner can be enormously helpful in keeping the indoor landscape free of temptation. Because a roommate sees you so much, he or she can remind you to practice the new eating behaviors you will be learning.

You may have a chubby roommate who wants to follow the program with you, but even a thin roommate can be a treasure.

Friends As Partners

I am using the word friend here to describe the people in your intimate circle. These are people to whom you talk regularly, in whom you confide, and with whom you spend leisure time.

A close friend who truly wants to help can be a superb

partner. Make sure he or she fits the guidelines and "passes" the test in this chapter.

You may even be able to form partnerships with *several* friends who want to lose weight with you.

Co-Workers As Partners

Even if you have a full-time partner at home, it helps to have a nine-to-five partner as well. Your work partner can close the door when the coffee wagon goes by, occupy you during morning and afternoon coffee breaks, go to lunch with you, and orchestrate celebrations when you lose weight.

Networking

Networking is the process of building an entire emotional support *system* of diet partnerships. Instead of one partner, you can have groups of supportive friends and relatives surrounding you in ever-widening circles. If you know more than one potential partner, take advantage of all this help!

Your inner circle of partners consists of the two, three, or four people who are closest to you. You may have a tight bond with one—a spouse, lover, or dear friend—but all of the people in the inner circle care deeply about your success.

Your middle circle consists of people who are important to you and whom you see regularly, although less often than your best friends. These are people you can call on when you need companionship and support.

Your outer circle consists of people you see less frequently and with whom you are less intimate. But they should be friends who will applaud you when you are successful on the program and will give you a boost when you may be having problems.

Your network of support people will see that you are never alone when you need warmth and friendship, and are never deprived of a compliment when you have done something to be proud of.

* * *

Here is the quiz I have designed to help you judge partnership candidates. Think each statement over carefully before you decide whether it is true or false.

There is no guarantee that a friend who "passes" this test will turn out to be an ideal partner. But it will certainly help weed out the definite "no-nos."

FRIEND PARTNERSHIP QUIZ

(check one answer for each question)

	True	False
1) It is easy to talk to my friend about my weight.	5	1
2) My friend has always been thin and doesn't understand my weight problem.	1	3
3) My friend offers me food when he or she knows I am on a diet.	1	5
4) My friend never says critical things about my weight.	3	1
5) My friend is always there when I need a friend.	4	1
6) When I lose weight and look more attractive, my friend will be jealous.	1	3
7) My friend will be genuinely interested in helping me with my weight.	6	1
8) I could talk to my friend about my diet even if I was doing poorly.	5	1

How to Score the Friend Partnership Quiz

Compute your score by adding the numbers that appear below each answer you chose. Compare your score with these ranges; then read the explanations that follow.

Score	Conclusion
30 to 34	This friend will probably make an excellent partner.
25 to 29	This friend may make a very good partner.
17 to 24	This friend is a questionable partner.
8 to 16	This friend is a very doubtful partner.

If you scored between 30 and 34, you may have found the perfect partner. A score in this range indicates that you and your friend are comfortable with one another and can probably follow the program with great skill.

If you scored between 25 and 29, your friend is potentially a good partner, but there are a few areas of concern. Try asking your friend to take the quiz and predict how you answered the questions. This may clear the air.

If you scored between 17 and 24, there are areas in which you and your friend may not be well suited as partners.

If you scored between 8 and 16, choose another friend who will be more supportive and helpful.

Do You Positively Need a Partner?

There is no question that you will find it easier to lose weight if you have a partner to work with you and encourage you. However, the weight-reducing program described in this book uses the best techniques science knows of to date. Your weight loss will be faster and smoother if you follow the complete Partnership Diet Program. But even on your own, it can be your most successful diet.

CHAPTER 3

The Partnership Process: Who Does What to Whom

How to Get Started

The first step: both of you sit down for a discussion. Here are some of the concerns you should talk about;

—Feelings about present weight
—What you see when you look in the mirror and when you look at each other
—What is motivating you to start the Partnership Diet Program
—What your family and friends have said or done in the past to be helpful
—Your feelings about beginning a program together
—How both of you will feel when the dieter reaches desired weight
—Whether you will diet together

The next step is optional but can be very helpful. Make a tape recording of your discussion about your weight, your weight goals, and the way you hope to feel when you reach your goals. Mention any specific feelings or incidents that make you want to lose weight. Put this recording away, to be brought out and replayed in the future when you need extra reinforcement to stay with this program.

For further motivation, take some pictures of each other

(you too, partner), perhaps in slacks or a bathing suit, and put them away with the tape.

As you progress through this book, you both will be learning dozens of behaviors and techniques for controlling your weight. Before you get to the specifics, you should both be aware of what your responsibilities are.

What the Partner Does for the Dieter

Partners, read this section carefully. It will start you on your way to fun and success.

1. *Partners Should "Model" Good Eating Habits*

Here's an example. One of the new eating behaviors for the dieter is putting the fork down between bites. This is an excellent way to eat more slowly (see Chapter 9), but until it becomes a firmly ingrained habit, it is easily forgotten.

A partner who also puts down his or her fork between bites does two good things for the dieter: he reminds the dieter to do the same, and he shows that he is really committed to helping that special person. Beware, however; your food will begin to taste better as you eat more slowly! If you aren't careful, you could become a real gourmet!

2. *You Should Keep a Daily Log*

You will be introduced to Daily Logs in Chapter 12, so I won't say much about them here. But it is important to know that "monitoring" the eating behavior of *both* diet partners is essential. What this means is that you will have a responsibility for recording how well you perform your new eating behaviors—and how well you are doing in the help-and-support department.

3. *You Can Reinforce Good Behavior*

Here is a basic principle of behavior:

> If a behavior is reinforced, it continues.
> If a behavior is discouraged, it stops.
> If nothing happens, it gradually fades.

Suppose the dieter remembers to put the fork down after every mouthful throughout an entire dinner. If you say, "That's great. You're really sticking with it. I'm proud of you," the dieter is likely to continue. If you say, "I wonder how long you'll keep it up? You never stuck with anything before," the dieter may give up in disgust. If there is no reaction at all, the dieter may be less and less conscientious about keeping up the good behavior, until it finally gives way to those old habits. My patients tell me that the importance of this *positive* feedback cannot be overemphasized.

4. *You Should Praise Behavior, Not Weight Loss*

Weight loss can at times seem very slow, so imagine how dreary it would be if your dieting partner received a compliment from you only when he or she lost a pound. There may even be times when the scale shows a weight gain instead of a loss, even if the dieter has been following the program exactly (see Chapter 14).

To make things worse, your partner may have to lose ten, fifteen, or even more pounds before people notice the slimmer figure and begin showering the dieter with compliments.

But if the dieter is praised for *behaving* appropriately, there will be many times during the day to earn the warm glow of a compliment. The dieter is entitled to praise for not buying snack foods at the supermarket, for eating slowly, for writing down the calorie count right after a meal, for eating half an English muffin at breakfast instead of a whole one. . . .

In one of my early groups for couples, Hank (the partner) was talking with Judy (the dieter). Hank was concerned about positive feedback. He said, "It is fine for me to help you by saying nice things, but I am making changes, too. I need that feedback as much as you do."

Hank was absolutely right. If his behavior change is to be continued, it must be rewarded, or at least acknowledged. Aren't you lucky? You will be getting some nice pats on the back also.

5. *The Partner Should Make a Big Production*
Out of the Weekly Weigh-In

Right now, at the start of the program, make a date—a specific day of the week and time of the day—for the weekly weigh-in. You should weigh *only* once a week, to make this a special event and to avoid watching day-by-day, ounce-by-ounce fluctuations. Your weight varies throughout the day, so always weigh at the same time.

Why such a big deal? Having a formal weigh-in *with*

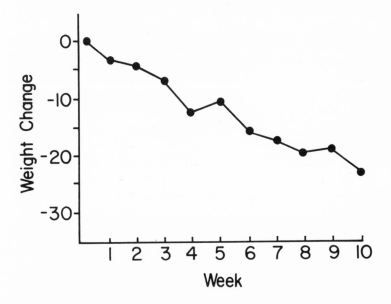

your partner is further evidence of how important your weight loss is to *both* of you.

Keep a record of your weight loss on a chart like this sample. If you are both dieting, use different-colored pencils for your dual records.

How to Help Your Partner Help You

Now here is the dieter's assignment—things you can do to make your partner an absolute genius at giving you the support you need.

1. *Make Specific Suggestions*

Requests such as "Please help me lose weight" or "Please be nicer when I'm trying to diet" aren't much help to your partner because they don't give clues as to *how* to help, or how to be "nicer." It is far better to say something specific and direct, such as, "Please eat your snacks in another room because seeing food makes me want to eat."

2. *Discuss How You Want to Be "Handled"*

Janet wanted her partner to be very strict with her. She told him to stop her if he saw her taking ice cream from the freezer or reaching for a second piece of bread. As she told her fellow dieters in one of my groups: "I want Harry to take the ice cream away, or at least ask me if I'm sure I have room for it in the day's calories."

Joan was horrified. "I hate being treated like a little girl," she said. "If Phil did that to me, I'd smack him. He should assume that I know what I'm doing. But I do like him to compliment me when I'm doing well."

It may take a little time for you to realize just what treatment makes you feel best. In the meantime, don't be annoyed if your partner is sometimes as confused as you are. If you work together, you will work it out.

3. *Reinforce Your Partner's Good Behavior*

If your partner does or says something that makes you feel good and helps you stay with the program, make sure you acknowledge it. Otherwise, those warm, supportive comments and helpful actions may cease.

You might say something like, "Thanks for clearing the table. It really helps when I don't have to face the leftovers." Or, "I'm glad we're taking walks together in the evenings. It helps me with the program and means a lot to me."

Since your partner may not be sure if a certain action or comment is helpful, be specific ("I like it when you compliment me for sticking with the program") rather than general ("Thanks for being nice").

4. *Ask for Positive Changes*

It is better to say, "It helps me when you avoid snacking in front of me," than to say, "You make it more difficult for me when you snack in front of me." There are usually two ways to phrase a request for help; try to think of the positive, rather than negative, way to do it.

5. *Do unto Your Partner as You Would Have Your Partner Do unto You*

As I have said, your partner can help you even without dieting with you. But if he or she does want to lose weight, remember that you have an obligation to help your partner follow the program, in the same way that you are being helped. Read yourself into the "partner" directions throughout this book.

The Psychology of the Partner

I learned a valuable lesson from my patients in my very first couples group. I asked the dieters what they wanted to accomplish during the program. Their first response was unanimous—and surprising. Their greatest desire was for their partners to *understand* their problem. One patient, Marilyn, said of her partner, "I know he means well, but he doesn't know how hard it is for me to lose weight and he has no idea how much I suffer because I am fat."

We concentrated on this issue during many of our sessions, and the partners *did* begin to understand the position of the dieter. However, it was not until Marilyn's husband,

John, spoke up that the obvious became clear: there were two people involved in this partnership, and the feelings of frustration were not just confined to the dieter. The partner had suffered, too. Before the Partnership Diet Plan can work, it is important for both parties to understand the feelings of the other. Ways for the partner to understand the dieter are presented later in the book. For now, I want to describe the feelings of the partner.

Here is a simple exercise that I use for each of my patients. Get a clear image in your mind of your partner and imagine yourself in your partner's position. Remember each diet and each of your periods of weight gain or weight loss. If you had been in your partner's position, how would you have responded? One dieter, Jeannie, explained, "I know it is frustrating to be with me when I diet. If I'd been in Herb's shoes I probably would have had *less* patience."

After many hours with my patients and their partners, I developed a scheme to characterize the psychology of the partner. There are three stages that most support partners go through in response to the dieter. Your support partner may be in any of the three stages. These are natural responses and they occur in the majority of partners I work with.

Stage 1: The Benevolent Approach. Most support partners want to help and start out with "nice guy" methods. If the dieter complains about weight, the partner may say something like, "Is there anything I can do to help?" or "You look fine to me." The partner may gently nudge the dieter to reduce and may even change his or her own eating patterns to assist the dieter. Yet the inevitable occurs and the dieter regains weight. This sends the partner to Stage 2.

Stage 2: The Martial Law Approach. When the nice approach fails, most partners declare "martial law." The dieter may be soundly criticized for overeating, the partner goes to great lengths to keep the dieter away from food, and the kind words come only after the dieter exhibits saintly vigilance. You won't be surprised that this doesn't work. The partner then moves to Stage 3.

Stage 3: Surrender. By this time the partner has exhausted the possible approaches and sinks into despair and resignation. The dieter's attempts to reduce are not taken seriously by the partner and there is no effort to help. The partner's frustration surfaces in sarcastic and angry comments.

DEVELOPMENT OF PARTNER ATTITUDES

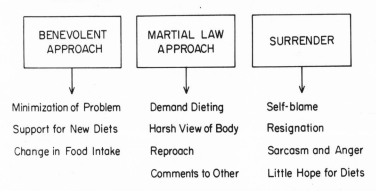

BENEVOLENT APPROACH	MARTIAL LAW APPROACH	SURRENDER
Minimization of Problem	Demand Dieting	Self-blame
Support for New Diets	Harsh View of Body	Resignation
Change in Food Intake	Reproach	Sarcasm and Anger
	Comments to Other	Little Hope for Diets

Since most dieters have been on dozens of diets, most partners are in Stage 3. At this point the partners and the dieter must be aware of two crucial facts.

1) Although most partners may not be aware of the feelings, they may feel that they somehow contribute to the problem and are deficient in not being able to help. Perish the thought! Overweight is a complex problem with many metabolic, biological, genetic, and psychological origins. Even scientists cannot determine the cause of a weight problem in a given individual, so the partners should not feel that they can blame themselves.

2) Even though the partner may feel that there is nothing he or she can do to help, nothing could be further from the truth. Read on!!

CHAPTER 4

Why You Can't Blow This Diet

Partnership Dieting Is Never Having to Say "Never"

Why won't I tell you exactly what to eat for breakfast, lunch, and dinner, from Monday through Sunday? Because it just won't work. Maybe it will for the first few days, while your motivation is still high. But with such an autocratic, restrictive diet, the first time you eat something that isn't on your food plan, you feel you have blown it. From there it is just a mouthful or two to guilt and helplessness—and another diet goes out the window.

Partners, this is good news for you, too. You must remember past diets where you and the dieter had to eat strange and unpalatable foods. You may have even been nice and eaten grapefruit every day! The Partnership Program will bring you and the dieter together, and eating will become even more creative and enjoyable.

On most restrictive diets there are too many "nevers"— cake, ice cream, corn on the cob, butter, milk, sometimes even fruit. There are usually too many "musts" as well. What if you don't like cottage cheese, get heartburn from cucumbers, or can't afford steak?

On the Partnership Diet Program you and your partner choose your own tasty, varied, nutritious meals—with lots of help from the recipes, menus, and calorie guides in the later chapters. You can live with *these* calorie boundaries!

What Is a Calorie?

Calorie counting is one of the basic and extremely effective techniques used in this program. It is terribly important for you and your partner to know what the numbers mean. Everyone is calorie-conscious these days. I hear things like, "That cake looks scrumptious. It must be loaded with calories." But a calorie isn't whipped cream or chocolate icing. What *is* it?

A calorie is the amount of heat needed to raise the temperature of one gram of water from 15 to 16 degrees centigrade.

That's not much help. Simply, calories are energy for your body. Everything you do requires energy—playing tennis, typing, watching TV, kissing. Even when you are fast asleep you are expending energy for your basic bodily functions.

The energy you use can be measured in calories: about 7 calories a minute playing tennis, 3 calories a minute doing office work, a little over 1 calorie a minute watching TV —or sleeping (see Chapter 11). The energy comes from the foods you eat; about 96 calories from a three-inch apple, 260 calories from a piece of cherry pie. . . . When food is utilized by your body, you get that amount of energy to spend on your activities.

How Are Calories Measured?

My patients are always curious about how we *know* that a cherry pie has more calories than an apple. Very simple— we burn it. The food to be measured is placed in a container called a calorimeter, which in turn rests in a larger container of water. When the food is burned, the temperature of the water rises. This increase translates into the number of calories in the food (at a rate, as I have said, of 1 calorie per one degree centigrade).

Obviously, the apple you eat may not be the exact size

of the apple burned by the scientists, so you can never know precisely how many calories you have consumed. Every apple is a bit different—and so are most calorie guides. But the charts are more than accurate enough for the purposes of your diet. And now that we are on the subject . . .

Why Are You Overweight?

You and your partner have your own theories about this. You both might be surprised by the other's thoughts about the cause of the weight problem. I hear a variety of reasons from my patients. Here are some of the most common:

"It's my glands." A few overweight people do have a glandular problem, but most only think they do, or would like to have that as an excuse. One or two of every hundred dieters may have a glandular disturbance; if so, it can be detected by a physician and should not be self-diagnosed.

"It runs in my family." Some dieters believe that obesity is hereditary. Science doesn't have all the answers yet, so we don't know the extent to which people inherit their weight problems. Even if overweight seems to run in your family, keep in mind that poor eating habits and underactivity are as likely to be passed along as "fat" genes.

"It's my metabolism." I often hear people say things like: "I eat like a bird yet I look like a rhino. My neighbor eats twice as much as I do and she's thin as a rail." Some people do seem to expend more energy than others; their bodies may be less efficient at utilizing energy, so they tend to burn more calories just *living*. Yet by and large, most overweight people simply consume more calories and expend less energy than their thin neighbors.

The REAL Reason You Are Overweight

The truth is, you are overweight because you have consumed more calories than your body needs. The excess calories are stored in your body as fat.

It's simple arithmetic: every 3500 extra calories that your body can't use become one pound of fat, stashed away somewhere on your person.

If your weight is stable, you are consuming just the number of calories your body needs to maintain its current weight. Your body fat is potential energy; it will just hang around until something happens to get it out of storage.

If you are in the process of gaining weight, you are continually storing up extra energy at the rate of one pound for every 3500 excess calories you consume.

You want to unload some of those pounds of fat, right? The way is clear: take in fewer calories than your body needs. Your fat stores will then be used for energy, and you will lose weight. If you simultaneously increase your energy expenditure by becoming more active, you will lose weight even faster. (Read all about *that* in Chapter 11.)

How Many Calories Should You Take In Every Day?

To estimate your body's daily energy needs, multiply your present weight by one of these numbers. The result will be the number of calories required to maintain your weight at its current level:

If you are:	Multiply your present weight by:
Extremely Inactive	13
Less Active than Average	14
Reasonably Active	15
Very Active	17
Extremely Active	21

How do you decide which category you belong in? Here are some guidelines:

Extremely Inactive. You indulge in no athletic activity, have a job requiring no physical exertion, and have a generally sedentary lifestyle (little walking, etc.).

Less Active than Average. You engage in athletic activity less than once each week, have a job that requires little exertion.

Reasonably Active. You engage in sporadic athletic endeavors (one to two times per week) and a moderate amount of walking, or have a job requiring exertion (lifting heavy objects or moving quickly) for five minutes at least three times each day.

Very Active. You engage in three to four weekly hour-long sessions of vigorous athletic activity (like running, swimming, cycling, handball, racquetball, etc.), as well as walking and using stairs daily. Or you are engaged in continuous and heavy physical labor for at least 40 percent of your workday.

Extremely Active. To fit this category you should be involved in extremely vigorous physical training, such as running at least one hour or ten miles each day (or the equivalent). Physical labor must be rigorous and must be continuous for at least 70 percent of the workday.

Discuss your assessment of your activity level with your partner; it is sometimes difficult to judge how active you are. Caution: an extremely inactive or athletic partner may over- or underestimate your activity level. If in doubt, get a second opinion. (Of course, these are guidelines and may not be totally accurate for every person; but they will serve our purpose very well.)

Here is a chance for both of you to dredge up those arithmetic lessons from grade school and to calculate your own energy balance equation. Based on our chart, a reasonably active 140-pound woman uses 2100 calories each day just to maintain that weight. The arithmetic: 140 pounds × 15 = 2100 calories. Suppose you are that woman, and you don't want to *stay* at 140 pounds.

Remember, for each 3500 calories you eat that your body doesn't need, you gain one pound; but if you take in 3500 less than your body needs, you lose a pound. Suppose you consume 1200 calories each day instead of the 2100 your body needs for maintenance. You will then be operating at a calorie deficit of 900 each day and in a little less than four days you should lose a pound.

What if you are a reasonably active 200-pound man? At 3000 calories a day you should neither gain nor lose weight. But suppose you reduce your intake to 1500 calories a day? In a little more than two days you should lose a pound. All things being equal, you could lose up to three pounds in a week. Beware though: most people are "less active than average" or "extremely inactive" and, therefore, require less energy.

Use these figures to determine your energy needs—and your partner's. This will show both of you how similar (or different) your calorie levels need to be. How do your figures compare with what you have been eating? I have used the numbers 1200 and 1500 deliberately. At 1200 calories a day, most women will lose between one and two pounds a week. At 1500 calories a day, most men will lose two or more pounds a week. These are the calorie levels I strongly recommend.

1200 Calories Each Day for Women— 1500 Calories Each Day for Men

You will find that you can eat comfortably and deliciously at 1200 or 1500 calories a day. If you have any doubt, take a quick look at the menus in Chapter 17.

Of course, you could lose faster by eating less—but one to three pounds each week is fast enough to give you a feeling of accomplishment. If you eat much less, you will be depriving yourself of foods you like and will be obsessed with food. If you are unhappy or uncomfortable, there is a danger that you may abandon the program.

Partners, take note—*your* expectations must be realistic. If you expect drastic weight loss, the dieter may feel compelled to make drastic changes. You both will suffer in the long run.

This calorie level may not be *exactly* right for you. In a few weeks you may find that you must cut back a little further before losing one or two pounds a week, or that you can afford to eat more calories and continue to lose. But use 1200 (for women) or 1500 (for men) as your initial guide and try to stay as close to your number as you can, every single day.

The Partnership Diet Program vs. the Others

Are you dreading the thought of deprivation? Look over this sample day with your partner and see if this looks like a diet. Notice the total calories for the day.

Breakfast

½ cup (4 oz.) vegetable juice cocktail	28
Cheese omelet (1 egg with 1 teaspoon grated Cheddar cheese cooked in a no-stick pan)	97
½ toasted English muffin, with	70
1 tsp. orange marmalade	17
Coffee with 2 tablespoons skim milk	11
	223

Lunch

¾ cup vegetable beef soup	59
2 oz. sliced bologna, on	156
1 slice whole wheat bread, with	59
1 sliced tomato, and	20
1 tsp. mayonnaise	34
¾ cup skim milk	66
	394

Dinner

Salad (6 Romaine lettuce leaves, ½ cucumber, 1 cut-up scallion), with	21
2 tbsp, diet Italian dressing	12
4 oz. lean T-bone steak, broiled	254
½ cup zucchini	12
½ medium baked potato, with	46

2 tsp. sour cream, and	16
1 tsp. chives	1
1 cup watermelon and cantaloupe chunks	45
Espresso coffee	—
	407

Snack

¾ cup skim milk	66
2 chocolate chip cookies	100
	166

TOTAL FOR DAY 1190

Any diet that allows you to eat English muffins, marmalade, mayonnaise, bologna, sour cream, potatoes, cookies, steak, can't be all bad, can it? If you were on a typical restrictive diet, or one of the popular "crash" diets that promise amazing weight losses in a week or two, you could have blown it by eating just *one* of these foods.

On a 1200-calorie or 1500-calorie regimen you have an endless variety of foods to choose from. Would you like ice cream instead of milk and cookies? Fine. Want corn flakes with fresh strawberries instead of juice and an egg? Terrific. See how easy it is?

But Maybe It's TOO Easy?

Audrey made this remark in her first meeting. "Being deprived is only natural on a diet and I feel guilty when I eat something that tastes good. What will keep me in line?" This is a common feeling. Some dieters can't adjust at first to the freedom of this program. They often have to work hard convincing their partners that they really *can* have all those delicious foods.

Are the following reactions familiar? And as for you, partner, do you believe these statements? "If I don't have a 'real' diet to follow, won't I eat all the wrong things?"

It is possible to be *under*nourished and *over*fed at the same time. As a "free agent" you must make a sensible adjustment between eating 1200 or 1500 calories of candy, cookies, ice cream, and black coffee, or the same amount of fruits, vegetables, milk, good protein, and grain products.

If your sweet tooth is what caused your weight problem in the first place, I suspect your initial reaction may be similar to Bea's: "The first three days I just went wild; a buttered bagel for breakfast, yogurt for dinner, and in between, only cookies and candy. I even lost a pound. By the fourth day I was starting to daydream about nice tart apples and juicy pears. Even the idea of cooked carrots and string beans was appealing."

By the end of the first week, Bea was eating sensible meals with the help of the nutritional guidelines I will give you later in this section. "I thought I would live happily ever after if I could just eat all the sweets I wanted without having to worry about my weight. I finally realized it was the *idea* of sweets I missed more than the taste. Now that I can allow for a piece of chocolate or cake anytime I want, it's not such a big deal."

"Won't I lose weight too slowly if I eat all that food?"

Most of my patients have had the experience of blitzing off five to ten pounds in a week on crash diets. They found that those big weight losses occur only at the beginning, when a lot of the loss is water weight. It rarely continues beyond the first couple of weeks, and usually happens to people who are quite heavy to begin with. (It is no trick for a 250-pound man to lose five pounds in a week on a strict diet.) Unfortunately, this weight tumbles back on nearly as fast as it fell off.

Here is the important point: *the more slowly the pounds come off, the more likely they are to stay off.*

"But I need someone to tell me what to eat!"

The "no-decision" feature of crash diets can be appealing. Aside from promising to melt ten or twenty pounds away in no time, many are totally structured, paternal, even dictatorial, and tell you exactly what to eat at every meal, every day. For some dieters it seems easier to have the same thing every day for breakfast, whether it's grapefruit and black coffee, toast and juice, eggs and water, or whatever.

Some people also feel better if they can look at Tuesday's menu on Tuesday and be told exactly what to have for lunch that day, even if it means eating foods they detest.

Some patients enter my program expecting that their partners will be telling them what to eat. In fact, some partners expect the same thing. As you'll see, the partner is a helper, not a manager.

Aside from the agony, the boredom, and even the danger of giving up in disgust, none of this prepares you for the real world—for a serious card game with your friends in the ladies auxiliary, or dinner at a Chinese restaurant with the office gang, or a snack at the Pizza Hut when you are shopping with the children.

On the Partnership Diet Program you and your partner can allow for any food event, anytime, anywhere.

Some structured eating may be helpful, especially at the beginning, before calorie counting becomes second nature and before you master the knack of eating a *little* of the foods you love instead of too much. For that reason, I have included an entire month of 1200- and 1500-calorie menus in this book (see Chapter 17). They are unlike other menus because they list, not only foods you cook yourself, but fast-food restaurant dishes and the frozen supermarket convenience foods that more and more singles and families are using these days.

Use my menus until you are comfortable working out your own meal plans. Sit down with your partner at the beginning of the week and plan seven days of menus from the lists I give you. Write out a master shopping list that either of you can take to the store. Assemble any recipes you need. That will be your diet plan for the week—far more exciting and delicious than any crash diet around. The beauty of this plan is that you and your partner can *both* find foods you love.

"Just because I tell myself I can only have 1200 or 1500 calories a day, what makes you so sure I'll do it!"

The numbers can't do it all by themselves. Even your partner, loving, helpful, and supportive as he or she may be, can't guarantee that you won't overeat. In the chapters to come you will learn how to count calories and how to recognize the situations, the people, even the thoughts, that send you out of control. You will practice dozens of techniques for coping with them.

You simply won't experience the same setbacks as you did on other diets.

Nutrition in a Nutshell

Your diet should fit your lifestyle, please your taste buds, and provide all the nutrition you need for good health. Now that you are losing weight, it is *especially* important to eat balanced meals. See how much your partner and you know about nutrition.

Nutritionists have different schemes for insuring a balanced diet. The most common, and the one you probably learned in school, consists of four basic food groups: Dairy Products, Fruits and Vegetables, Breads and Cereals, Meats and Protein.

For the Partnership Diet Program I have separated fruits and vegetables into two categories, to make meal planning easier. This simplifies planning for calories. For most people, eating a specified number of servings from each of the following five food groups will ensure a reasonable diet:

1. *Dairy Products.* This includes milk and milk products, e.g. yogurt, ice cream, and ice milk. Remember that skim milk has fewer calories than whole milk, and ice milk

fewer calories than ice cream. (By one serving I mean 1 cup milk or the equivalent.)

2. *Vegetables.* This includes all fresh and frozen vegetables. Certain vegetables are very low in calories and can, therefore, be eaten as desired. These include asparagus, broccoli, cabbage, cauliflower, celery, cucumbers, eggplant, green beans, kale, lettuce and other leafy greens, summer squash, and spinach. Have a green, leafy vegetable every day and a yellow vegetable every other day. (One serving = ½ cup or one medium, e.g. tomato.)

3. *Fruits.* This includes all fresh, frozen, and canned fruits and fruit juices. Have fruit (orange, grapefruit, strawberries, melon, etc.) every day. (One serving = ½ cup sliced or cut-up fruit or juice, or 1 medium-sized fruit, e.g. apple, or half a large fruit, e.g. grapefruit or banana.)

4. *Breads and Cereals.* This includes whole grain or enriched breads and cereals, pasta, rice, dried beans. (One serving = 1 slice of bread or 1 ounce of a packaged roll, bun, or muffin, or 1 ounce of ready-to-eat or uncooked cereal, or ½ cup pasta, rice, etc.)

5. *Meats and Proteins.* This includes meat, poultry, fish, peanut butter, cottage cheese, and Cheddar cheese. (One serving = 1 ounce.)

The precise number of servings you should have every day from each category depends on several factors. Nutritional needs differ among people, and you can satisfy your body's requirements with many different combinations of foods from the five groups.

What *are* your body's requirements? The Food and Nutrition Board of the National Academy of Sciences National Research Council has established these guidelines: for the *average* adult, the Recommended Daily Allowance (RDA) of carbohydrates is 125 grams, and the RDA of protein is 40 grams. Here is a list of the average carbohydrate and protein grams supplied by one serving of each of the five food groups:

	Carbohydrate	Protein
Dairy Products (1 cup)	12 grams	8 grams
Vegetables (½ cup)	5 grams	2 grams
Fruits (½ cup)	10 grams	0 grams
Breads and Cereals (1 slice or ½ cup)	15 grams	2 grams
Meat (1 ounce)	0 grams	7 grams

You can consume the RDA for carbohydrates and proteins in a variety of ways. These hypothetical diets are just two of many possible combinations for a single day's eating.

Food Group	# of Servings	Grams of Carbohydrate	Grams of Protein
Example 1			
Dairy Products	3	36	24
Vegetables	2	10	4
Fruits	2	20	0
Breads and Cereals	5	60	10
Meats	1	0	7
		Total 126	45
Example 2			
Dairy Products	1	12	8
Vegetables	4	20	8
Fruits	5	50	0
Breads and Cereals	3	45	6
Meats	3	0	21
		Total 127	43

The two examples are very different from each other—but each has adequate carbohydrates and protein. This shows how you can maintain good nutrition but still remain flexible in your eating.

The following are guidelines for maintaining a balanced diet:

Adult Nutritional Guidelines

Food Group	Servings Per Day
Dairy Products	3–5
Vegetables	3–5
Fruits	2–4
Breads & Cereals	3–4
Meats & Potatoes	1–2

These guidelines are appropriate for most people. Dietary requirements vary with age, sex, activity level, and other factors. There are special requirements for pregnant women and for people with certain medical conditions. Maintaining a balanced diet is essential for good health, and you should consult your doctor if you have special nutritional needs.

The Partnership Diet Maintenance System

There will come a day when you look at yourself in the mirror and say: "That's it. This is the weight I want to be."

You will know how you got there, but will you know how to stay there?

You *already* know.

Let's assume you are a reasonably active woman and you want to maintain your weight at 120 pounds. Remember how you calculated your energy needs? Do the same for your new weight: $120 \times 15 = 1800$ calories.

Doesn't that sound terrific? An additional 600 calories a day . . . half again as many as you were eating on the program. But these numbers are not set in stone. First, these mathematical formulas are not 100 percent accurate. It is possible that the best maintenance level for you will be closer to 1700 or 1600 calories, not 1800. Second, your body has grown accustomed to the amount you have been feeding it and may not adapt well to many extra calories. Third, weight loss can change your metabolic rate, so at a lower weight you may need to multiply your weight by a lower number.

My patients have found that the best way to determine their own maintenance level is to add 100 calories to the daily allotment at first and stay at that level for at least one week. Then add 100 more calories for another week. If you are still losing weight, you are below your maintenance level. If you change the rate at which you expend calories (through activity), you will have to adjust your food intake.

You know the techniques. *You* are in control.

You and your partner are about to begin seven of the most eventful days you may ever know. You will learn the principles of Partnership Dieting and will learn the plan for permanent weight loss.

PART 2

The Seven-Day Course in How to Eat, Think, and Act like a Thin Person

In this section you and your partner will learn the techniques that make the Partnership Diet Program so effective. You will learn to combine forces to work on a shared goal.

This section can be mastered in seven days. It is designed so you can read a new chapter each day. You will acquaint yourself with new behaviors for one day, and then you will move on to a new topic. After you have covered each of the areas, I will give you a timetable for implementing your new habits into a lifetime pattern of weight control.

CHAPTER 5

Day One–How to Keep a Diet Diary

Today you will learn a behavior that may be the most important in the book. What could be so important? *Recording the food you consume in your Diet Diary.* This simple procedure will take no more than five or ten minutes each day and will make you and your partner experts on eating habits. You will learn to take control of your eating.

The Diet Diary serves two purposes, both of which concern the partner. For the partner, you will learn all about the dieter's eating patterns, and you will be able to determine the role of these patterns in the dieter's problem. The diary will motivate the dieter to eat less, so it is important for you to encourage conscientious record keeping. I will teach you how to do this as we move along.

To begin, write down every single thing you eat or drink, along with its calorie count, on the form that I have included in this chapter. (You won't have to buy a calorie book to do it. The Appendixes contain *the* most comprehensive calorie guide available anywhere.)

Before the day is over, make sure you get a small notebook for your permanent Diet Diary to keep a record of each day's calories. You may want to make photocopies of the form so you have one for each day, or you may prefer to have a handy notebook.

For day one, don't change how much you eat, how often

you eat, or what you eat. This will be difficult because you are motivated to change, but you need this information to construct your program. Simply record everything.

You and your partner may be surprised at what today's diary reveals. Are you far from your calorie goal? Do you eat more often than you thought? Do you skimp on some meals, only to overindulge at others? Do the calorie counts of some of your favorite foods shock you?

In just one day you will begin to see how helpful your Diet Diary will be. It will accomplish seven supremely important things for you:

1. *Your Diet Diary Will Teach You Everything You Always Wanted to Know about Calories but May Have Been Too Full to Ask.*

Do you feel virtuous when you snack on hard cheese or cottage cheese? One ounce of Swiss or Cheddar or American cheese contains more than 100 calories. Cottage cheese goes for 90 to 120 calories per half-cup serving. What about that handful of potato chips? Ten of those little chips contain 110 calories—nearly 10 percent of a 1200-calorie allotment.

Most of my patients are amazed at calorie totals. Their partners are even more surprised if they have never had to worry about weight and consider calorie counts. The more you and your partner know about calories, the easier it will be to regulate the waistline.

Once you become familiar with calorie counts, you will enjoy delicious snacks at no more (sometimes less) than the cost of so-called diet foods. For example, you can tear into half a cantaloupe filled with a half-cup of blueberries for just 105 calories, or enjoy three ounces of shrimp with a tablespoon of tangy chili sauce for just 93 calories.

2. *Keeping the Diet Diary Is the Only Way for You (and Your Partner) to Be Aware of Exactly What You Eat*

Some of my patients think their meal patterns are much different from what they actually are. Jennifer thought her eating was confined to three meals per day. A look at her diary showed a different picture.

a) Jennifer had breakfast: orange juice, cold cereal with milk and a sliced banana, and coffee with milk and sugar.

b) She nibbled two slices of salami and a chunk of cheese while she made her sandwich for work.

c) At the office Jennifer had her usual coffee and buttered roll.

d) At lunchtime she ate her sandwich, then went out to do some errands, bought a candy bar, and ate it on the way back.

e) She had a soft drink in midafternoon when someone sent out for Cokes.

f) She had dinner with a friend after work: a Bloody Mary, lasagne, two pieces of Italian bread with butter, a glass of red wine, black coffee.

g) She and her friend shared a box of buttered popcorn at the movies.

h) She had a glass of milk and some cookies while watching the late news.

From her diary Jennifer discovered that the salami and cheese, the candy bar, and the Coke *alone* had contributed 330 calories to her day's total. She admitted that if she hadn't recorded these snacks, they would have been lost from her memory.

Most of my patients have eating amnesia; it is easy to "forget" some of what you eat or drink; the peanuts you absent-mindedly munch with a drink, the bread you eat before the waiter takes your order, the meatball you "taste" while you cook a spaghetti dinner. . . . A little forgetfulness is natural. However, you may *want* to forget. There is no way to be fooled if you write in the Diet Diary conscientiously after every meal or snack.

3. *The Diary Will Raise Your Consciousness*
   about Your Eating Patterns.

Keeping your Diet Diary will make you aware of problem areas. Business lunches may be more loaded with calories than you realized. Perhaps you plan to eat only one meal each day and you can't understand why you don't lose weight.

Margaret's day one diary spotlighted her problem instantly.

Every day was the start of a new diet for Margaret. She had a cup of black coffee "to get my heart started" in the morning, lunched on a piece of fruit, and by dinnertime

DIET DIARY

BREAKFAST

Food	
Coffee black	0

Total Breakfast Calories   0

LUNCH

Apple, small	70

Total Lunch Calories   70

DINNER

Meat Loaf, 4 slices	340
French fries, 20	310
Lima beans, 1 cup	180
Apple pie, 2 pieces	750

Total Dinner Calories   1580

SNACKS

Cheese, 1 oz.	105
Saltines, 8	98

Total Snack Calories   203

Total Calories For Day   1853

she was so hungry she could have eaten her way through the table leg. She then ate a huge dinner and a bedtime snack. When she started recording her calories, Margaret realized that her "one meal a day" amounted to more calories than she was entitled to for the entire day.

Can you spot similar self-defeating habits in your own diary?

4. *The Diet Diary Puts You in Control of the Whole Day's Eating.*

Alice was keeping her diary for the first time. After dinner she added her calories and found that she was just below her allowance for the day. She then decided to sip a cup of tea rather than eat a piece of cake. She was proud of herself and probably would have eaten the cake if she hadn't been keeping the diary.

5. *You Can "Bank" Calories for a Special Occasion.*

Going out to dinner tonight? By keeping track of your calories throughout the day, you can save as you go along, in order to "afford" the garlic bread or the chocolate mousse you know you will want at dinner.

6. *Your Diet Diary Will Help You to Lose MORE Weight.*

This is the clincher: my experience has shown that those dieters who are the most conscientious about keeping records are the ones who lose the most weight!

7. *The Diet Diary Gives the Partner Information about the Dieter's Progress.*

This part of the program can be thoroughly enjoyable and can bring you closer together. The diary is an instant and reliable record of the dieter's progress. The scale may not always show the progress even if the dieter has had superb control over eating. In these cases, the dieter needs some self-satisfaction and the partner needs to know that the dieter is actually doing well. The diary provides this information.

Now that you are convinced of the importance of your Diet Diary, here are some guidelines to help you keep track of calories with Einsteinian accuracy. There are a number of ways both of you can work together on these.

1. *Don't Guess: Look Everything Up.*

In the beginning, don't assume that you know, remember, or can guess the calorie value of anything. Look it up. For the support partner, you can become a calorie expert by looking up the values of foods and by helping to figure the calories in complicated cases. You both will memorize the counts for foods you have regularly, like your morning juice or toast, the milk in your coffee, and the apple you have for a snack. Your calculations will be lightning fast.

2. *Record Immediately after Eating.*

If you wait until the end of the day, you are likely to forget some of the things you ate, and even if you remember, you may be hazy about the amounts. When you are tired and ready for bed, it is hard to recall whether you had eight or twelve potato chips with your sandwich at lunch, or whether you had three or four ounces of fruit salad. Whip out your diary and record what you ate as soon as the last mouthful disappears from your plate. If you are rushed, write down the amounts and tally the calories later.

The partner can help here by reminding the dieter so nothing escapes the diary, and by carrying an extra diary in case the dieter forgets it someday. You can aid the dieter by being supportive during the initial stages where record keeping is just beginning.

3. *Don't Leave Anything Out.*

Never say, "Oh, that doesn't count." Every calorie counts, and nearly everything has calories—including the mayonnaise on your sandwich, a bite of a friend's apple, a stick of chewing gum . . .

4. *Weigh and Measure Everything.*

A kitchen scale is indispensable. If you don't have one, it should go to the top of your shopping list. If your birthday or a holiday is near, your partner may want to give you a scale as a gift to emphasize its importance. (Don't be shy about hinting.)

It is important to weigh foods that are dense in calories, like steak or hard cheese, where a small mistake can make a big difference. Even after you train your eye to be pretty accurate at estimating, you should still make a practice of weighing everything. For example, don't just pour cold cereal into a bowl and slosh milk over it. Weigh the cereal, then pour the milk from a measuring cup to keep track of how much you use.

A practiced eye will be helpful in judging restaurant portions, but don't hesitate to ask. In any decent restaurant the waiter should be willing to weigh your portion of steak or bluefish if you request it.

What about home-cooked meals? Any dish with several ingredients (like a beef stew) should be handled this way: count up the calories for each component (vegetables, meat, any canned ingredients like beef broth, tomatoes, etc.), divide the finished dish into equal serving-size amounts, and divide the total number of calories by the number of portions. Keep your own serving separate. Store leftovers in single portions, and remember to tape the calorie count to the container.

Measurements are as important as weight. The cantaloupe half listed in my calorie guide (see Appendix) is not the same as half of a monster melon you buy at a country fruit stand; adjust your count accordingly.

5. *Review the Diet Diary Together Every Day.*

At the end of the day (or whenever you two get together), go over the diary. Put your heads together and look for patterns and problem areas. If you are both dieting, compare notes for the day. For the dieter, don't be shy about showing your diary to your partner—it will get easier. For the partner, don't be critical, and remember that the *very act* of completing the diary is a major step. Here is an example of a working partnership:

One of my patients became known as "the popcorn lady" after she told her Partnership Diet group this story: "Ralph noticed from my diary that the biggest problem in my day seemed to be the coffee wagon at the office. He knows I'm mad for popcorn so he suggested that I bring unbuttered popcorn to work each day. Now instead of getting something sweet from the wagon, I bring out the popcorn. My boss thinks I'm nutty, but it works."

Compare the calories in a cup of *unbuttered* popcorn— about 25—with the calories in the average *plain* Danish pastry—about 275—and you may become a popcorn person yourself!

DIET DIARY

Name   Date

BREAKFAST   Food

Total Breakfast Calories ——

LUNCH

Total Lunch Calories ——

DINNER

Total Dinner Calories ——

SNACKS

Total Snack Calories ——

Total Calories For Day [   ]

The preceding is a day's page from the Diet Diary. You may want to draw up your own page or make copies of this. Be sure that the form is easy to use. Many of my patients buy a pocket-sized notebook and transform it into a diary. This way they can look back over past days.

Supporting Each Other

You both know that this program involves changes for the partner. Your eating patterns (and ways of dealing with each other) have taken years to develop. Therefore, changes may not come easily for either of you. Remember that we all respond well when nice things happen.

It is important for you to support each other by doing nice things. At the end of this and the next six chapters, I will list ten supportive things you can do for your partner. You can probably think of more, but use these for starters.

It is common at this point for my patients to think that these suggestions are for the partner so he or she can support the dieter. This is only partly true. The partner needs support also, and what better person to provide it than the dieter? If you are the dieter, think of using some of these methods to reward your partner for being so helpful.

Supportive Strategies for One or Both Partners

1. Send a love letter
2. Balance the checkbook
3. Buy a handsome leather-bound or fabric-covered book to serve as an elegant Diet Diary
4. Make a date to watch a sunset
5. Buy a record
6. Clean out the garage or basement
7. Buy a set of wildly attractive sheets for the bed
8. Get tickets for the opera, a play, or a ballgame
9. Make Sunday breakfast
10. Offer to give your partner a massage

6

Day Two—Taking the Mystery Out of Eating

Are there places where you always snack? Do certain moods —boredom, depression, elation—start you snacking? Do some people inspire you to overeat? You and your partner may have discussed these possibilities; what did you decide?

The foods you eat may be strongly influenced by where and when you eat, with whom you eat, what you are doing, and how you feel. If you can zero in on these influences, you can learn to eliminate them, work around them, or cope through some response other than eating. You can take firmer control by penetrating some of the mystery that surrounds your eating. Today you and your partner will learn a technique that can help you do just that.

The form shown here is similar to the Diet Diary but has been expanded to include information about the circumstances of each eating episode. Use this form instead of your Diet Diary today, to start learning more about your eating behaviors.

Some of my patients enjoy guessing beforehand what the extended diary will look like. They are often surprised. Partners may also be surprised if they try to guess what the diary will show.

It isn't likely that you can pinpoint every troublesome area in just one day. (The timetable in Chapter 12 allows for extended use of this special diary.) Today you will be-

DIET DIARY

	Food	Time	Place	People	Feelings	Activity	Calories
BREAKFAST							
						Total Breakfast Calories	_____
LUNCH							
						Total Lunch Calories	_____
DINNER							
						Total Dinner Calories	_____
SNACKS							
						Total Snack Calories	_____

Name ___ Date ___

Total Calories For Day [ ]

gin to learn about the people, places, times, moods, and activities that seem to trigger eating. Here are some danger signals and ways to deal with them. In the chapters that follow you will learn even more techniques for handling these problems.

When You Eat

Do you snack all evening when there is nothing better to do? Perhaps mornings are a problem—when it's just you and the washing machine. Or maybe your co-workers can set their watches by your four o'clock journey to the candy machine. Once you spot these habitual eating times, start to work derailing your eating urges.

Buy an engagement calendar. You and your partner fill

in two or three evenings a week with away-from-home activities. If it isn't possible to go out, make at-home "dates" to mount all your photographs in an album . . . play Master Mind or Monopoly . . . hook a rug . . .

Perhaps you and a neighbor can take turns doing your laundry together in one house or the other. How about arranging to do the most interesting parts of your job between three thirty and four thirty, to keep the candy machine out of your thoughts?

Where You Eat

Whoever invented dining rooms and kitchen tables probably never dreamed that modern man could figure out so many other places to eat:

On the platform (at the bus stop), waiting for a train (bus)
On the train (bus)
In a parked car
In a moving car
Walking down the street
Standing by the back door
At your desk
At a co-worker's desk
At the kitchen counter
In the laundry room
In bed
In a beach chair
In the den, living room, bathroom, basement, garage . . .

Make a list of the three (or more) places where you do most of your away-from-the-table eating, and start to dissociate food from those spots. Partners can speed this process along in many clever ways. One of my patients awoke one morning to find that while he was sleeping his wife had taped a NO FOOD ALLOWED sign to the headboard of their bed.

What Else You Do while You Eat

If you watch TV while you eat—or eat while you watch TV—the television has probably become an eating signal for you. The first step in unlinking this pair of behaviors is to become aware of the association; there is more help in Chapter 7.

Do you have a kitchen phone with a cord that conveniently reaches the refrigerator or the cookie jar? Some of my patients have removed the kitchen extension so they make calls from a location where food is less accessible. Shortening conversations is also a help; some of my patients use kitchen timers to set limits on their phone calls.

Search your diary for other activities that you tend to link with food: reading the morning paper, studying, doing a crossword puzzle, waiting for the dishwasher to stop . . .

With Whom You Eat

Do you eat more when you are alone or with friends—with certain people but not others? One patient reported that she could keep calm during her weekly visits to her mother only by eating steadily as soon as she arrived at her mother's house. Her solution: "I take her shopping or to an art exhibit. We're away from the kitchen, and she just can't get to me as badly when we are out doing something."

Another patient realized that she did most of her serious eating with her friend Burt. Overweight but unconcerned, Burt devoted entire evenings to eating at Italian or Chinese restaurants, and Ginny found it difficult to resist keeping pace. She tried to talk Burt into going for a light snack and then a movie, but he preferred the restaurants. Ginny finally decided to stop dating Burt, at least until she had her own eating habits under control.

How You Feel When You Eat

These are some of the moods and feelings we all experience from time to time:

Happy	Worried	Uneasy
Content	Depressed	Restless
Neutral	Angry	Frustrated
Tense	Pressured	Bored
		Tired

The feelings are universal, but the responses to them can vary. Which feelings prompt you to eat? You may not consciously say, "I'm angry because I didn't get the raise I expected, so I think I'll console myself with an ice cream sundae." Or: "I'm so happy I got that raise, I think I'll have an ice cream sundae to celebrate." But the feeling somehow translates itself into the action.

Keeping your diary will help you see connections between food and mood, so you can start to look for non-edible ways to respond. For example, instead of cooling your anger with ice cream, you could check the Help Wanted ads and start looking for a better job. Instead of topping your raise with hot fudge and a cherry, you could celebrate with tickets to a play for you and your partner.

After you have completed the new diary, analyze your results with your partner. Have a thorough discussion about what you find because upcoming chapters will teach you ways to change your eating patterns.

Prerecording—Coping with Difficult Situations

As you and your partner become experts at recording and analyzing your eating behaviors, a variation of the recording procedure may be helpful. Instead of eating and then recording, record first, then eat. Some of my patients find this to be an extremely powerful technique. In one controlled experiment, dieters who recorded before they ate lost more weight than those who recorded after they ate. You may find this helpful if you reach a plateau with your weight or if you don't feel you are losing fast enough.

How does it work?

Suppose you are having roast beef, mashed potatoes, and broccoli for dinner. Slice your portion of meat, weigh it, look up the calorie count, and write it down. Do the same with the vegetables. Then decide whether you are going to have bread with your meal and, if so, how much. If you are too full to eat some food when the time comes, you can always cross it out. Angel food cake for dessert? Slice it and record it.

If you decide to have a snack, let's say an apple and a piece of cheese, don't just hack off a hunk of Edam. Cut it, weigh it, write it down. If the calorie count turns out to be higher than you thought, there is still time to take a smaller piece.

In restaurants, check the menu and decide what you want, from first course to an after-dinner beverage. Tell your partner, or anyone you are eating with, what you have decided—to make it official. Write down the choices in your Diet Diary along with their calorie counts. Now you can order—but only one course at a time. You may decide to have less than you planned.

Why does it work?

1. Prerecording gives you a powerful incentive to eat only what you have written down. When you do, there is a feeling of real accomplishment. Every meal and every snack can be an occasion for you to feel good about yourself. It can also be a signal for praise from your partner.

2. Prerecording helps you avoid unpleasant surprises. By now you may have memorized the calorie counts for all sorts of foods and snacks that you eat regularly. But occasionally you can be in for a shock if you wait until after you eat to look up the count. Finding that a Big Mac has 540 calories instead of the 300 or so you guessed can be sobering.

When you do know, you can make an informed decision: is there room for a Big Mac in your day's calories, or should you choose a Filet-O-Fish (400 calories) instead? Or can you only afford a cheeseburger (306 calories)?

3. You are less likely to indulge in spur-of-the-moment extras. Let's stay at McDonald's for the moment. Once you decide on a Filet-O-Fish and black coffee, you are less likely to add an order of French fries (regular, 210 calories) and a vanilla shake (325 calories) at the last minute.

Prerecording puts you in *control*, not helplessly at the mercy of a tempting smell, or what someone else is having, or a picture on a counter card, or other environmental eating cues.

4. Prerecording can help you limit automatic eating. Want some potato chips? You know they contain 11 calories each. How many can you afford? You decide on twelve, write down 132 calories in your diary, take twelve out of the bag, put the bag away, *then* sit down and enjoy the chips. I suspect potato chips have never tasted so good! Without prerecording you might have poured some chips into a bowl and eaten your way through them automatically without even thinking about how many you were having— until the moment of reckoning.

5. Prerecording is another means of using the Partnership approach. Kristie and her friend Paul used prerecording when dining in restaurants. Kristie would decide what she wanted and would record her choices while discussing the calories with Paul. Paul would then order meals for both of them. It was a joint process that each enjoyed.

Supportive Strategies for One or Both Partners
1. Buy a nice plant
2. Plan a surprise birthday party
3. Send a "congratulations" telegram
4. Fix something around the house
5. Buy a hardcover book, so your partner won't have to wait for the paperback
6. Polish the silver

7. Buy extravagant cologne or perfume
8. Give a gift certificate for something special
9. Do the food shopping for a week
10. Do part or all of the Christmas shopping

CHAPTER 7

Day Three—Protecting Your Eating Environment

Are you hungry right now? If the answer is "yes," how do you know? Are you hungry because it is time to be hungry, because you are doing something that makes you hungry; or do you feel some physical sensation like a gnawing feeling in your stomach? Perhaps you feel hungry because you aren't full. There are many cues that people use to determine whether they are hungry. Ask several friends and your partner how they know they are hungry. Believe it or not, most people never think about it.

If you eat only in response to physical signals of hunger, you might not have a weight problem. But a study by Dr. Albert J. Stunkard, of the University of Pennsylvania, has demonstrated that people who are overweight often eat when they are not hungry—that is, when they are not getting *internal* signals of hunger. People who are not overweight tend to eat in response to real hunger pangs, but overweight people respond to many *external* eating cues as well.

Times of the day, people, places, and activities can be cues to eat. So can the mere sight of food. Consider this: the average child sees 10,000 food commercials on TV each year. It's no wonder many of us grow up with a sensitivity to food. (The wrong foods, too; did you ever see a commercial for celery or carrots?)

It will show you and your partner how to eliminate some of the eating cues from your environment. First, take this quiz to find out how responsive *you* are to environmental eating cues.

This chapter is especially important for partners. There are many ways you can help alter the eating environment, but it may not be easy if you are also tuned in to those signals. Take the quiz to see how responsive you are compared with the dieter.

WHAT'S YOUR ECQ*?

(*Eating Cue Quotient)

Check "yes" or "no" for each of the following questions. Compare answers with your partner's to see which situations are troublesome.

	YES	NO
1. I sometimes keep on eating even after I feel full.	____	____
2. I often get hungry when I watch others eat.	____	____
3. I get an urge to eat when I see a delicious dessert, or when I smell good cooking, even if I have just eaten.	____	____
4. There are certain times of day when I almost always feel like eating.	____	____
5. When I pass a bakery, a pizza parlor, or any other place with delicious food, I want to stop and eat something.	____	____
6. I nearly always eat when I do certain things, like watch TV or read the morning newspaper.	____	____

7. Seeing pictures of delicious foods in
   magazines or on TV makes me want
   to eat.   ____   ____

8. I almost always eat everything on
   my plate.   ____   ____

Did you answer "yes" to question 1? Then you may not
be paying enough attention to what your stomach is telling you. To keep eating after you feel full is one sign that
your internal signals are being overruled by external cues.

Did you answer "yes" to one or more of questions 2
through 7? If you get an urge to eat from the sight of a
luscious cake or a sizzling steak, the smell of pizza or freshly
baked bread, even a picture in a magazine or a completely
non–food-related activity like reading a paper, your environment is exerting a strong influence on your eating
habits.

If you answered "yes" to question 8, you are being influenced by the amount that is served, not by what your
body needs. This can lead to trouble in several situations.
Some restaurants pride themselves on serving oversized portions. But you don't have to eat it all. The people who love
you may try to feed you to show how much they care. But
they can learn to show their love by feeding you *less*. Even
when you serve yourself, there are probably times when you
portion out more than your body wants. Haven't you sometimes said, "My eyes were bigger than my stomach"?

It's time to take control of your eating behavior. You
can do it by learning four new habits that I will discuss in
this chapter. You will need time to make them part of your
life (see the timetable in Chapter 12), but you can start
working on them with your very next meal.

Leave Some Food on Your Plate at Every Meal

My patients tell me that leaving food on their plate is
the most difficult of all the new habits, and also one of the
most helpful.

Were you taught as a child to "clean your plate"? Did you have to sit at the table until your plate looked as though it had been through the dishwasher? Did you go without dessert until you had eaten everything else? Were you told that you couldn't play with your friends or watch your favorite program until every speck of food was eaten, because of "all those children starving in . . ."?

If you learned the "clean-your-plate" habit, you were not eating what you needed, but what somebody else *thought* you needed. You were at the mercy of the server. Unfortunately, this habit is so firmly ingrained in many overweight people that they feel compelled to eat whatever is on the plate no matter who puts it there—even themselves.

It is important to break this habit, so you eat only what you need. Eating all of the food on your plate means that you are eating in response to an external cue: food on your plate.

Leaving some food on your plate reminds you to respond to an inner cue (hunger) rather than an external cue (the sight of food). It will help increase your awareness of internal hunger signals by forcing you to decide whether you are still hungry. This will interrupt the automatic eating that usually proceeds until your plate is clean.

Begin right away by setting aside a small portion of food on your plate. This is *not* an exercise in eating less: it is practice in being conscious of how much you are eating and how much you really want. The act of setting aside some food is more important than how much you set aside. Robert and Jean made a game of this by seeing who could leave aside the smallest portion. Robert thought he won the contest with one lima bean, but Jean managed to leave one half of a pea!

Partner, here is a good place for you to help. If you leave some food on your plate you will remind the dieter to do the same. The power of "modeling" will be evident when you do this. In addition, you will be showing your support

through your actions. Don't worry about starving! Even if
you take more than one serving, be sure to leave a little at
the end of the meal. If you find this hard to do, you will see
how difficult it is for the dieter to make changes in long-
standing eating behaviors.

Start out by setting aside a portion of the food you like
least. When you can do this comfortably, start leaving aside
small portions of other foods and of side dishes as well. You
will be a master of this behavior when a tiny portion of each
food is left over. If you feel it would help to increase the
amount you leave aside, do it in a gradual fashion.

Don't starve yourself. Your goal is to break a habit (eating until you have emptied your plate) and to replace it
with a new habit (eating only until you have had enough).
Eventually you will no longer have to set aside some food
at the beginning of the meal, because you will automatically
stop eating when you have had your fill.

Are you worried that leaving food over is a waste of
money? During this phase many of my patients find clever
ways to avoid throwing food out. Maurice mixes it with the
dry dog food he feeds his collie. Sally requested a food processor from her husband-partner for an anniversary gift and
uses it to make soups from the leftovers for her next day's
lunch. (See "Cream-of-Anything Soup" in Chapter 16.)
Even if you and your partner do throw a little food away,
you are not really being wasteful. Think of the cost of gaining weight: new clothes, medical bills, possible heart sur-
gery . . . !

You have seen that the mere presence of food on your
plate can be a powerful eating cue. But that's not all. Any
time of day, any place, any activity that you associate with
eating can also become an eating signal.

Eat at the Same Time Every Day

Do you snack in the afternoon or at bedtime just because you are accustomed to this practice? Do you tell your-

self, "If it's six o'clock, I must be hungry"? Do you eat un-
planned snacks on impulse, or skip a meal and then more
than make up for it later?

If you eat at certain times because of habit rather than
hunger, you are almost sure to take in more calories than
you need. What's worse, you are not in control of your eating life.

The remedy: plan an eating timetable for every day,
and stick to it. Include snacks as well as meals on your
schedule.

In a sense you are making eating "dates" with yourself
and your partner. Schedule breakfast, lunch, and dinner.
Plan a coffee break at the office, a midafternoon snack at
home, or whatever fits best into your day. Just make sure
you allow for these snacks in your daily calorie allotment.

The eating timetable is something that can be profitable
for both the dieter and the partner. Plan some of the meals
together. This will enhance the effect of the support that
takes place between you two and will make for structured
times of enjoyment.

Partner, your role in this is to be available as much as
possible for the scheduled mealtimes. Even more impor-
tantly, you should confine your eating to scheduled mealtimes when you are in the dieter's presence. Remember that
the dieter may be prone to eat in response to the sight of
food, and you can be very helpful by removing this signal
at times when the dieter is not scheduled to eat. You might
be able to go even further by encouraging others in the environment to do the same. This might include other family
members, friends, co-workers, etc. It may be hard for the
dieter to ask these people for help, so a kind word from you
may do the trick.

Why is an eating timetable so important? If you know
exactly when your next meal or snack is planned, you will
be less likely to eat beforehand. If you plan specific eating
times and eliminate random nibbling, you will limit the

times of the day you associate with eating. There will be far fewer times when the hands on the clock can trigger an eating response.

Always Eat in the Same Place

If you eat wherever you happen to be—in bed, sitting at your desk, standing at the kitchen counter, on the train or bus—then these places can become associated with food and can signal you to eat. If you want to break those associations, limit the number of places in which you eat.

Pick a certain spot in your kitchen or dining room and eat only in the chosen spot. Be as specific as you can, down to the place at the table and the chair that are yours alone, just for eating. Don't eat anywhere else, and don't do anything else in your eating place. Each meal should be a special event, not confused with other activities. If you eat in the same restaurant, cafeteria, or luncheonette quite often, try to sit in the same area each time, if possible at the same table. You might even do what one of my most successful patients did. Claudia bought a colorful flowered placemat and napkin for her own use at home—and another set to take with her and use when she ate out at her favorite restaurant.

What if you eat at your desk? *Don't* eat at your desk. Find another spot at work where you can quietly open your brown bag—the corner of a co-worker's desk, the lounge, or simply another part of your own office. If you habitually eat at your desk, you will associate food with a place where you spend a great deal of time, and it will be hard to break the habit of eating there. Even coffee breaks should be taken away from your desk.

Here is another place for some partner assistance. You, partner, can help by eating in the same place as the dieter and by avoiding putting pressure on the dieter to eat elsewhere (in front of the TV).

Do Nothing Else while Eating

Have you ever finished a whole bag of potato chips while watching a TV program, or eaten three donuts with your morning coffee while reading a newspaper?

For you, sitting down in front of the TV set or settling down with a book or newspaper may be a cue to eat. When these associations between food and other activities become firmly fixed, you are likely to eat even though your body is not physically hungry.

The antidote: make eating a *pure* behavior. When eating, don't do anything else. No TV watching, reading, studying, sewing, talking on the phone, crossword puzzles. . . .

It is perfectly acceptable to talk with your family and friends while eating, or to have some soft music playing in the background for company if you are alone. In fact, you may find that your discussions are more enjoyable because you aren't distracted by other activities.

When you do nothing but eat while you eat, you eliminate the automatic eating that often takes place while you are doing something else. You enjoy your food more, because you concentrate on tasting and appreciating it, without distractions. Also, you are reinforcing the habit of responding to your *internal* cue to eat when you are hungry, not an external signal to eat just because you are doing something you associate with food.

Partner, you can be an important stimulus for change. You can help the dieter resist temptation to do other things by making lively conversation at your planned meals. Ed helped Marie with this by learning a new joke or some funny story each day. Even though Ed was a miserable storyteller, Marie was amused by his effort and thought her meals were more fun as a result. If *you* are accustomed to watching the news or reading the paper while you eat, this may be a difficult sacrifice for you to make. It will go a long way in helping the dieter, so you can be a useful supporting cast by making these changes and by encouraging others to do the same.

Supportive Strategies

You and your partner have probably found some clever ways to support each other for making important changes in your eating habits. You can have a tremendous influence on each other, but you have to *do something* (it doesn't happen magically). Here are ten more suggestions about rewarding each other:

1. Offer to pay for a long-distance call to a dear friend
2. Do the laundry for a whole week
3. Buy a clock radio so your partner can wake to music
4. Plan a mystery weekend and make all the arrangements
5. Find a lovers' lane and have fun
6. Buy a pocket calculator—to count calories
7. Offer to see a movie your partner wants to see but you don't
8. Order a singing telegram
9. Telephone at an unexpected time and ask for a date
10. Place an ad in the classifieds and say something nice about your partner

Day Four—Dealing with the Three Main Food Danger Zones: Shopping, Storing, Serving

Today you will learn to deal with three primary danger zones: shopping for food, storing food, and serving food. You and your partner are about to learn methods to wrest control of your eating environment from those food signals that can be so troublesome. As you both read these next sections remember this battle cry:

Out of Sight, Out of Mouth!

Because the mere sight of food is enough to make many overweight people eat, removing food from view—and learning to deal with food when it can't be ignored—can really aid in your efforts to reduce.

Is your home booby-trapped with visible edibles? You and your partner are about to become the Food Vice Squad! Go through the house and remove food from every room except the kitchen. This means taking candy and nut dishes from the living room, confiscating the chewing gum and candy that lurks in the bedroom, and banishing pretzels, potato chips, and dips from the family room. You may even want to deputize other members of the household to help with this task. This will show them how important it is to abide by this simple rule: Keep Food Out of Sight.

In my clinics I find that partners become more and more animated when we discuss this topic. Even before we discuss specifics, they tend to think ahead of how they can help with these danger zones. If you feel the same, your enthusiasm is well founded because there are many ways you can help. In one group Lennie spoke up and said, "I have always wanted to help Claire, but I never knew exactly what to do. I am amazed at how many ways I can help with food cues. It makes me feel like I am doing something."

Let's go to work. We will start with one area that can lead to real progress.

Shopping for Food

You can gain greater control over the food that enters your house by following the guidelines I will give you in this section. If you can exercise good judgment when you buy food, you will not be faced with so much temptation later, when the food is beckoning to your hungry taste buds. It is easier to lose weight if prudent food choices are made *before* you are confronted with the signals that tend to break down your resistance.

In this chapter, the partner will have a corresponding assignment for each assignment for the dieter. Discuss which behaviors are applicable for your partnership situation and then carry on!

1. *Shop Only after You Have Eaten.*

You know what it is like to shop when you are famished. Beth explained this to her group: "When I am hungry I buy tremendous amounts of fattening foods, all of which I want to eat immediately. When I get home I eat much more than I should, and I always have a lot left over that I feel obliged to finish. Sometimes I feel guilty enough to throw the bad foods away, but usually I eat them within one or two days."

Be sure to shop on a full stomach. You will feel less inclined to make impulsive purchases, and you won't be faced with the presence of food later. If you cannot schedule shopping trips after a meal, eat something low in calories before you go (perhaps a cup of tea and a lettuce and tomato salad).

Partner: Some partners in my clinics have taken over the food shopping from the dieter. This, of course, leads to great control over the food that enters the house, as long as the partner makes wise selections. Lennie and Claire traded tasks. Lennie agreed to do the food shopping each week if Claire took care of the lawn in the summer and shoveled the snow in the winter. Claire liked the switch because she could get some exercise in the yard and because she wasn't faced with the problem of choosing foods.

This approach is fine, as long as the new shopping patterns can be permanent. If the dieter ultimately will be doing the shopping, it is best to learn coping strategies as soon as possible. One way of doing this is to shop together. You and the dieter can invent methods of conquering the high-calorie temptations that line some of the aisles. Shopping can become a leisurely and enjoyable event where you can both brainstorm about food combinations that will promote weight loss. If this isn't possible, be sure to encourage the dieter to shop after eating.

2. *Shop Only from a List.*

Plan out a list of items before you go shopping and after you have eaten. It is best to plan the list with your partner, to take only enough money to buy the items on the list, and to avoid buying foods that you have not planned to buy.

Partner: Work with the dieter to make a shopping list. When you shop with the dieter, practice buying things from the list, and see if you can avoid aisles that do not contain foods that are on the list.

If both of you are dieting and you don't live together, go shopping together. Trade lists and shop for the other's food.

You can switch baskets at the check-out line. What better way to make sure your basket has the right food? At the very least, call each other and compare lists, then discuss what you actually purchased later.

3. *Avoid Shopping with Children.*

Children have lightning-fast reflexes and can fill your cart with sugar-coated cereals, cookies, and candies faster than you can maneuver the cart. The check-out line is particularly dangerous. Notice how the candies are at eye level for children? You are busy removing items from your cart, people behind you are in a hurry, and the last thing you need is a scene created by a child who is denied a candy bar.

Partner: Take care of the children while the dieter shops. If you shop together, entertain the kids so they won't fill the cart with goodies. Better yet, this may be an excellent time to start training the kids about nutrition and proper eating. Spend some time in the fruit and vegetable sections and try to get the kids excited about these healthy foods.

4. *Buy Your Least Favorite Snacks.*

There are times when you must buy foods for others. If chocolate chip cookies are your weakness, buy fig bars or macaroons. If you hate cheese crackers but love pretzels, buy cheese crackers. This also applies to foods that you must have around for your family, perhaps for the children's lunch. You would be surprised at how well the family can change the types of food they snack on; but if some problem foods must be around, buy ones you don't prefer.

Partner: When you bring home foods for snacking, smuggle them in as though they were Christmas presents. If possible, buy or request foods that the dieter does not like.

Note: Remember that you can eat anything on the Partnership Diet Program. The techniques in this chapter are to help you modulate the *amount* of food you are exposed to and to help prevent automatic and compulsive eating when you aren't really hungry. Denying yourself something you really like is counterproductive. One of my patients, Sarah, said this recently: "I love this program because I can have ice cream every evening. I have a small portion and still keep to my calorie goal. On other programs where ice cream was forbidden, I would be so nervous that I would either binge on ice cream and feel guilty or I would quit the program."

Storing Food

Some people eat food for the same reason Sir Edmund Hillary climbed Mount Everest: because it's there. You and your partner can do many things to reduce the number of times you are exposed to food. Here are some ploys for keeping out of harm's way by keeping food out of *your* way.

1. *Store Food in Opaque Containers.*

Brownies in a glass jar can't help but be enticing. The same goes for other foods you can't resist. Use metal canisters, coffee cans—anything you cannot see through.

My patients have devised clever ways of accomplishing this. Margie recalled, "I have a handsome collection of old canning and apothecary jars, and they used to be filled with candies, cashews, and cookies. I emptied them all last week and filled them with imported teas, coffee beans, dried herbs, and pasta." These foods are all handsome, but are not the stuff binges are made of.

Partner: Think of some innovative ways to keep tempting foods out of the dieter's sight. If you have problem foods around the house, be certain to keep them stored where they can't be seen. For example, potato chips can be removed from the bag and stored in a plastic container.

2. *Store High-Calorie Foods in Out-of-the-Way Places.*

Even though your cookies may be in an unmarked tin, they may be trouble if they are too easy to get. Put those foods on the highest shelves or behind other items in the top cupboards. One of my patients put all the high-calorie foods in the basement on a high shelf. "I know the foods are there, but I no longer grab at them compulsively. And if I do eat them, I get a little exercise going to the basement and using the stool to reach them!"

Partner: Help the dieter by storing your food in out-of-the-way places. You might also take charge of locating the places for the dieter's food, so the dieter has even less inclination to eat automatically.

3. *Keep Harmless Foods in the Front of the Refrigerator.*

Seductive foods should be tucked neatly behind cans, bottles, or anything else that can obscure your view. Keep fresh fruit and the vegetables you like up front so you are lured by low-calorie treats. You might even unscrew the refrigerator lightbulb so your food doesn't look quite so glamorous!

Partner: Conduct periodic inspections of the refrigerator to make sure that low-calorie foods are most visible. Do some rearranging if you find the situation merits your attention.

4. *Freeze Foods that Tempt You.*

Freeze anything that you can get your hands on. Although some of my patients will even eat a frozen bagel in a pinch, the time necessary to thaw most foods will limit compulsive eating. Also, if the piece of cake is frozen and you take the time to thaw it, you must really want it and should go ahead and have it. But remember the old saying, "A watched cake never thaws!"

Partner: If you have a stash of high-calorie foods that will last more than a few days, freeze most of it and unthaw portions at a time. If the dieter digs in, only a modest amount can be eaten at any one time. Of course, this isn't necessary for foods that do not entice the dieter.

Serving Food

You have maximum contact with food when you are preparing and serving it. Restraint becomes difficult because you must be in contact with the food. There are, however, several methods you can use to remain in control. Your partner can be very helpful with these behaviors, so be sure to plan your attack together.

1. *Remove Serving Dishes from the Table.*

The Pennsylvania Dutch are famous for their family-style meals—platters are laden with food and do not leave the table until the feast is over. This can be hazardous for someone with a weight problem. If the food is there, it is easy to be tempted into eating more than you need.

Put casserole dishes, meat platters, and serving bowls back in the kitchen after serving. Ask others to help themselves if they want extra servings. If you get the desire for another serving, you will have time to reflect on how much you have eaten and whether you are physically hungry. Some of my patients ask their partners to serve the second helpings to control portion size.

Partner: Is it possible for *you* to serve food at meals? This will be a great help to the dieter because contact with food will be minimized. After everyone is served, you can remove the serving dishes to the kitchen. If you want second helpings, avoid asking the dieter to get them for you. You might be surprised to know how much you can influence the dieter's eating with this simple step.

2. *Clear Leftovers Directly into the Garbage.*

When your meal is finished, bring the plates directly to the kitchen and put the scraps into the garbage. If possible, bring the waste container into the dining room and scoop the remnants of food right in. Remember, the sight of food can make you feel hungry, even if you aren't. In one of my recent groups Denise admitted, "I am embarrassed to say this, but I found from my Diet Diary that I consume plenty of calories after the meal is over, when I clear the table." She was surprised when three other members of the group said they had the same problem. You can make this task easier by imagining you are taking fat from your hips and discarding it into the trash.

Partner: If you do not usually clear the table, take command! This will further decrease the dieter's contact with food. If you and the dieter have a household division of labor, you can have a big impact by taking over some of the food-related chores.

3. *Leave the Table Immediately after Eating.*

The longer you are exposed to the sight and smell of food, the easier it is to feel that you are still hungry. You can prevent this by removing the serving dishes from the table—or by removing yourself from the table. Try to leave the table when you finish eating so you don't linger around the food. If you finish before everyone else, consider the possibility that you are eating very fast. If so, Chapter 9 will be particularly useful.

Partner: Assist in this new initiative—to leave the table after eating. If you usually have coffee or tea after the meal, clear the table first and then adjourn to another room for beverages and pleasant conversation. Dinnertime interactions are important to many families and partnerships. See if they can take place away from food.

4. *Eat Everything from Dishes, Not Containers.*

Even if you are alone and you are just having a small snack, do not eat from containers. Put crackers in a small bowl, cottage cheese on a plate; even fruit can be sliced and eaten from a plate.

Eating from containers can have two untoward consequences. First, you may eat automatically without paying attention to what you are eating. This cuts down on the pleasure you get from each bite of food. Second, eating from the container obscures the amount you are consuming. Peanuts or pretzels on a plate will seem more satisfying than the same amount eaten from a jar or a bag.

Partner: You can model this behavior by eating all your food from dishes when you are with the dieter. When you two are having a planned snack, avoid eating from containers.

5. *Use Smaller Utensils.*

In a recent experiment, two groups of overweight people were served the same amount of food, one group on salad plates and the other on regular dinner plates. The dinner-plate people did not report being satisfied, while more than 70 percent of the salad-plate group did report being satisfied!

Use a salad or luncheon plate instead of a dinner plate, a juice glass instead of a water glass, a bouillon cup instead of a soup bowl, a teaspoon instead of a tablespoon, and a dessert fork instead of a meat fork. This will slow the rate of eating and will make you feel satisfied with less. My patients report that this increases the enjoyment of food.

Partner: Be a model citizen and use smaller utensils while eating with the dieter. *You* might even begin to enjoy your food more!

6. *Serve Yourself One Portion at a Time.*

If you want two pieces of toast, prepare one and eat it before toasting the second. If you want a whole container of cottage cheese, take a small portion and put the container away before eating it. Even if you are positive that you will be back for more, take one serving at a time.

This will help control automatic eating and will give you an opportunity to decide how hungry you are along the way, not just at the beginning. If you prepare two pieces of toast, you will probably eat the second even if you are not hungry. By preparing one piece at a time, you may surprise yourself and forgo the second.

Partner: If you are doing the serving, assume the dieter wants a small portion, and eat small portions yourself. You do not have to eat less, just use smaller servings. If you and the dieter are at a restaurant, order the courses one at a time. This will slow the meal and will give the dieter time to determine whether he or she is still hungry before each course.

7. *Avoid Being a Food Dispenser.*

Are you the one who dishes out meals, packs lunchboxes, hands food around at parties, buys the food for office functions, or picks up snacks for co-workers? The more contact you have with food, the more often you will be overcome by temptation. Ask a co-worker to get the snacks or to procure the food for the office parties. If you have your own cocktail party, see if a friend will help with the preparation or serving. Think of other ways to avoid dispensing food.

Partner: Take over some of the food dispensing chores. If you are having a party, help with the handling of the food. Pack the childrens' lunchboxes, or teach the older ones to do it themselves. Many kids realize they are helping the dieter by doing this and are proud that they can make their own lunch. If someone must be the "gatekeeper"—the person who controls access to the food—tell the dieter you are taking over the exalted position.

Reminder

I have given both of you many new behaviors and there has been little time to practice them. When you reach Chapter 12, there will be a timetable to follow so you can practice these new habits until they become permanent behaviors.

My patients feel that each new behavior is fun to use initially, especially when undertaken in the cooperative spirit of Partnership Dieting. The novelty will diminish, and you both must stick to your new behaviors with Herculean determination. Here are more methods for supporting each other along the way:

Supportive Strategies
1. Buy a fine wine for your partner
2. Leave an "I love you" note somewhere where your partner will find it
3. Get an enlargement of your partner's favorite picture
4. Defrost the refrigerator
5. Buy a single place setting of beautiful china, so even the lowest-calorie meal is elegant
6. Collect travel brochures from your favorite places
7. Plan a dream vacation, even if it is a fantasy one
8. Give your partner first choice of which TV station to watch
9. Buy a book of photographs or art works
10. Get a wok, so your partner can make low-calorie vegetable dishes

CHAPTER 9

Day Five—Eat Slower and Enjoy Less Food More

Would you qualify for a gold medal if the Olympics had a speed-eating event? Some of my patients eat very fast, while others eat no faster than the thin people they dine with. No matter which group you belong to, learning to slow the rate of eating can speed your rate of weight loss.

You and your partner may think that slowing the rate of eating will be tantamount to halting a runaway freight train, especially if you are used to eating meals as if you are running a fifty-yard dash. But there is plenty each of you can do. Best of all, you can do it together.

Your Stomach Has No Taste Buds

Today I want you to begin eating a new way: slowly. My patients are sometimes skeptical when I say that slowing eating will lead to decreased caloric intake and *increased* enjoyment of food. How can this be?

Eating Slowly → Fewer Calories

Appetite and satiety (feeling full) are very complex physiological phenomena. One way to view the process is to imagine a feedback loop that connects your stomach and your brain. When food reaches your stomach and intestines, it is broken down so the nutrients can enter the bloodstream. A message is then transmitted to the brain indicating that nutrients have been absorbed, and you feel full. Research has shown that this process takes approximately twenty minutes.

When you eat very rapidly, the message doesn't reach your brain until you have stockpiled more than your body needs. This explains why people often say, "I'm stuffed—why did I eat so much?" By slowing the rate of eating, you allow this message to be transmitted *before* you have overeaten. You feel just as satisfied, but with less food.

Eating Slowly → More Enjoyment

As you begin to eat more slowly, you will savor your food rather than ingest it mechanically. The food will have longer to tantalize your taste buds. You will enjoy particular tastes, and you will have time to notice subtle combinations of flavors and contrasts in textures. Herbs and spices will become more evident and you will appreciate how they blend together. Two of my patients, Peg and Sharon, became real believers after they slowed their eating.

Peg ate enormous quantities of nuts, particularly peanuts and cashews. When I had Peg record how much pleasure she experienced from eating these foods, she was surprised that she was tasting very little of what she ate. "Now that I eat more slowly I am getting tremendous pleasure from the nuts. I have been combining peanuts, cashews, raisins, and dry cereals to make a delicious mix. I like to take bites with my eyes closed so I can pick out the individual tastes. I know the mix is high in calories, but I eat much less now."

Sharon was much the same. "I used to think that lasagne just tasted like lasagne. Now that I take my time I can taste the different flavors—the creamy cheese, the tangy sauce, and the spicy sausage. I eat only about half of what I used to, and the same has happened with other foods."

Putting the Brakes on Eating

When I reach this point with my groups, my patients greet me with a resounding chorus: "I have been eating this way all my life. How can I change now?" The answer is simple.

The rate at which you eat has been learned over many years. You probably learned from your parents. Perhaps you raced through meals so you could play with friends, or maybe you developed your habits at school, gulping down food in a noisy and crowded lunchroom. If we filmed your eating in many situations, we would find remarkable consistency in your eating rate, even if we made precise measurements like the number of bites per minute.

Your eating rate is a firmly ingrained pattern. But just as you acquired your present style, you can acquire a new style. You and your partner can use the following procedures to lower the speed limit on your eating.

1. *Put Down Your Fork between Bites*

This is a very effective way to decelerate your eating. When you take a bite of food, place your fork on the table and pretend it is anchored there until you have chewed and swallowed the food. The same procedure applies to finger food like toast, a piece of fruit, or a sandwich. Take a bite, put it down, chew, and swallow, then pick it up for another bite.

Partner: Put your fork down between bites when you eat with the dieter. Many of the dieters in my groups have trouble with this behavior, not because it is so difficult, but because they forget to do it. If you are setting a good example, there is a double chance that the dieter will follow through. The dieter will also appreciate this visible sign of your interest. The partners in my groups often report that *they* begin to enjoy their food more, because they pay more attention to tastes. I'll bet you didn't expect such a bonus when you began this program!

Both of you may feel awkward when you first attempt this procedure. Perhaps you will experience what Hal did. "Since I was putting my fork down between bites, I had a chance to observe how thin people eat. They take a bite, put down their fork, talk to the person they are eating with, pat their lips with a napkin, move some food around on their plate, butter a piece of bread and put it down without taking a bite, and other things that I thought would make me look funny."

2. *Pause During Each Meal*

Sometime during each meal, take a break and relax. Start with a thirty-second break, then gradually increase the time until you are comfortable with a three-minute pause.

Partner: Take the break with the dieter. You may wish to be the official timekeeper for the pause. You can also be inventive and devise things to do during the break. You might quiz each other on the day's news events, have a trivia contest, make a pass (you can accomplish a lot in three minutes!).

Why do I tell my patients to "call a time-out" during each meal? The pause allows you to huddle with your teammates (your stomach, taste buds, and brain). After careful consultation, you can decide exactly how hungry you are. Your stomach will have time to notify your brain that you have eaten. Recent studies with animals show that interrupting a meal leads to decreased food intake even if the animal is given free access to food after the pause.

If your meals are family affairs, the pause may transform the dining table from a place of heavy eating to an arena for light conversation. Sallie uses the dinnertime break to sponsor a joke competition among her three teen-age sons. "Each has one minute to tell a joke, then we vote for the funniest joke. The winner gets a round of applause. We all enjoy it and the kids like the attention." Sallie keeps a three-minute egg timer on the table. It is a nice reminder to take a break and it keeps track of the time.

You may worry at times that your hot meal will become unappetizingly cold while everyone is telling jokes. You can avoid this by pausing during a dish that will not suffer from the delay. The best times to break are just before or just after the main course. If you start a meal with juice or soup and make a separate course of the salad, you can schedule your pause after you finish the salad. You can also break between the main course and dessert.

3. *Limit Liquids at Meals*

When my patients begin to pay close attention to the way they eat, many say they miss the full enjoyment of food by washing it down in a stream of liquid. By limiting your liquids at meals you will enjoy your food more and eat less in the process. You need fluids in your diet, but it is fine to have them before or after the meal. In fact, prefacing your meal with a large glass of water, diet soda, mineral water, iced tea, or other low-calorie beverages can give you a sensation of fullness even before you start the meal. You may want to have a cup of tea before dessert rather than with dessert.

You and your partner can make a regular practice of having a no-calorie cocktail before or after the meal. The partner can help during the meal by limiting liquids and thus slowing his or her rate of eating.

When you cut down on liquids, you will increase how much you chew your food. This prolongs the time that food can massage your taste buds. Also, liquids aid in the digestive process, so if you decrease your liquids you will feel full with less food.

4. *Be the Last Person to Start and Finish Each Course*

When you are eating with other people, talk, rearrange your napkin, cut your meat into tiny pieces . . . stall any way you can to be the last person to start eating. During the meal maintain a pace that will guarantee that you are the last one finished. This exercise will help you slow your eating. Of course, if you and your partner are both dieting, you will have to take turns finishing last, or you may never finish your meal!

Breaking the Eating Chain

You and your partner have learned many techniques for weight control; you will learn many more. Specific procedures are useful, but you are faced with the problem of deciding which procedures to use and when to use them. If you learn the principles of behavior, you will be able to make accurate decisions in all eating situations. This is true of any science, like physics, for example. To determine the maximum speed an object will attain when dropped from the Empire State Building, the physicist will apply a principle (a mathematical formula) to the specific situation. One important behavioral principle is chaining.

Any eating episode, even an impulsive snack, takes place at the end of a long series of behaviors. This series is like a chain, and every step is a link. Each link is necessary for the chain to lead to the final behavior (eating).

Here is an example of how one such chain (with eleven links) can lead to a seemingly casual act: snacking on cookies. You and your partner go through this example and discuss the techniques you have learned to deal with each link of the chain.

You go to the supermarket (1) on an empty stomach (2) with no specific idea about what to buy (3). As you stroll through the aisles you spot your favorite cookies (4) and decide to buy them (5). When you get home you take the cookies out of the grocery bag and leave them on the kitchen counter (6). Later in the day you are watching television and begin to feel hungry (7). You wander into the kitchen (8) and see the cookies on the counter (9). You want to get back to the television, and since the cookies are right there and ready to eat (10), you grab a handful and eat them (11).

You could have broken the eating chain at the very end, by showing superhuman restraint and leaving the cookies. But the last link is the hardest to break. Let's use your new skills to analyze the situation and to break each of the eleven links in the chain.

(1) The cookie confrontation could have been avoided altogether if you'd let your partner do the shopping. You could have gone shopping with your partner, or if you and your partner were both dieting, you could have traded carts.

(2) If you had to do the shopping yourself, you could have eaten first and then shopped in a less vulnerable state.

(3) Shopping from a list would help screen out high-calorie snacks. Making the list with your partner would have been like investing in cookie insurance.

(4) Strolling casually through the aisles of a super-market can be trouble. Markets are planned so staples are tucked away on high or low shelves, but high-calorie goodies are right at eye level, in flashy packages. Shop in a market you know, and go straight to the items on your list. Ask the manager instead of wandering up and down the aisles looking for certain items.

(5) The chain could be broken by purchasing something other than cookies. Cookies aren't forbidden on the Partnership Diet Program, but buying them should be under your control, not under the control of external cues.

(6) By leaving the cookies on the counter you are sowing the seeds of temptation. Store the cookies in an opaque container, place the container on the highest shelf in the kitchen, or freeze the cookies.

(7, 8) Does the television make you hungry? Instead of heading for the kitchen, turn your back when the food commercials come on. Use the time to knit or to do stretching exercises. Make sure you avoid eating while you watch TV to break the association with hunger. Put a bowl of carrot sticks, radishes, and cauliflower on the counter instead of cookies, so your initial view will be of low-calorie foods.

(10) Buy cookie mixes instead of packaged cookies. This will limit impulsive eating and you will get more exercise mixing the batter than opening a package.

(11) If you decide to have cookies, put them on a plate (one at a time), go to your designated eating spot, and do nothing else while eating.

Supportive Strategies

1. Plan a trip to a museum
2. Get a new board game
3. Start a photo album or a scrapbook
4. Plan to pick your own fresh fruit—strawberries, cherries, blueberries, etc.
5. Get a puppy or a kitten.
6. Get wood for the fireplace
7. Make popcorn in the fireplace
8. Make a special gift (hook a rug, knit a scarf, etc.)
9. Send flowers from "an admirer"
10. Arrange for a sitting with a professional photographer for "after" pictures

CHAPTER 10

Day Six–How to Think Yourself Thin

In one of my recent groups I had an interesting conversation with one of my patients, Rosemary, and her partner, Arnie.

Dr. B.:	What is the single most important factor that determines whether you succeed or fail on a diet?
Rosemary:	My attitude. Usually it stinks.
Dr. B.:	Why does your attitude play such an important role?
Rosemary:	If I have a positive attitude, I can stick to any diet, but I always start feeling negative and then I lose control. It happens on *every* diet.
Arnie:	If she gets down on herself, it's all over. There's no way to convince her that she might do well.
Dr. B.:	Rosemary, how important is *Arnie's* attitude?
Rosemary:	If Arnie has a positive attitude, I feel much better. But when I start to get negative, he gets frustrated and then I feel even worse.
Arnie:	I get upset because there is nothing I can do.

For both the dieter and the partner, attitudes can be a great friend or a dangerous foe. Rosemary and Arnie expressed the feelings of many dieters and their partners. They made one thing very clear.

Your Thoughts Can Be Fattening

Our minds are continually filled with thoughts, feelings, and emotions. We feel good about our accomplishments and bad about our shortcomings. Most dieters are under constant attack from their own thoughts. These thoughts can be changed. Today you will start thinking like a thin person.

The first step: take the Dieter's Attitude Quiz to diagnose your fattening thoughts. Look it over with your partner, then read on for my interpretation of your answers. Assessment of the partner's attitudes will follow.

DIETER'S ATTITUDE QUIZ

	Agree	*Disagree*
1. Once I cheat or binge on a diet, I might as well quit.	___	___
2. To be successful I must not compromise on the foods I should eat.	___	___
3. I am rarely satisfied with what I accomplish.	___	___
4. No matter how well I do, I feel I should have done better.	___	___
5. There are some foods I must never eat if I want to control my weight.	___	___
6. A successful dieter can resist temptation at all times.	___	___
7. I have less will power than most people.	___	___

8. Some people are naturally fat, and I am one of them.   ____   ____

9. It seems unfair that some people never have to worry about their weight.   ____   ____

10. Sometimes I feel I have been unjustly treated by God or Nature.   ____   ____

What are some other negative thoughts you have? The quiz contains only the most common; my patients generate dozens more. If you agreed with any of these statements, or if you have similar thoughts of your own, you are harboring destructive attitudes that can be important obstacles to your efforts to reduce. Fear not! You are about to become a positive thinker.

Diet thoughts fall into specific categories. Correcting the negative thoughts is possible if you follow my guidelines. I will give you the guidelines shortly, but first, here is the diagnostic key to the quiz.

If you agreed with questions 1 or 2, you probably feel you are either "on" or "off" a diet—the light bulb mentality. The smallest transgression sends you "off" the diet; you then feel inadequate and say things like, "What's the use anyway?"

Questions 3 and 4 help identify dieters with the "impossible dream" attitude. You can inadvertently maneuver yourself into a negative attitude by setting overly ambitious goals. Many dieters set goals that *nobody* could reach.

If you agreed with questions 5 and 6, you are a victim of the "awful imperatives"—inflexible rules that are out of touch with the realities of daily living. Questions 7 and 8 point to the "dead-end thinking" that can make you give up in despair before you give yourself a fighting chance. Finally, questions 9 and 10 show that some dieters have a "wishful thinking" attitude that can interfere with the businesslike conduct of a weight-loss program.

Partner Attitudes

Partner: Your role in this program is important, and your tasks are not easy. A simple fact demonstrates how crucial your role can be—research has shown that dieters do better with partners than without partners. You are learning ways to change *your* eating patterns and ways to change how *you* eat when you are with the dieter. This requires motivation and genuine commitment.

Partners in my groups are forceful in their claim that attitudes are important determinants of how effectively they can assist the dieter. With a positive attitude you can help a great deal, but it may be harder to help when the negative attitudes set in. Let's examine some typical partner thoughts in the Partner's Attitude Quiz. Then I will show you and the dieter how to shrink the waistline with positive thoughts! Check the statements that apply to you.

PARTNER'S ATTITUDE QUIZ

	Agree	*Disagree*
1. When the dieter eats fattening foods, I feel like he/she blew the diet.	——	——
2. If I think about it, I expect the dieter to be perfect all the time.	——	——
3. Sometimes I feel like I have contributed to the dieter's weight problem.	——	——
4. When I try to help the dieter and there is no weight loss, I feel I have let the dieter down.	——	——

5. The dieter has a weight problem because of a lack of discipline and will power.   ____   ____

6. If the dieter loved me enough, he or she would lose weight.   ____   ____

7. There are some foods the dieter should *never* eat.   ____   ____

8. When I think of the dieter's weight problem, I sometimes think there is no hope.   ____   ____

Which of these statements reflect your thoughts? Are there others that are more appropriate to you? Look back over the categories of statements for the dieter's attitudes to see which apply to your thoughts. Do you have unrealistic goals for yourself or for the dieter? Are you one to throw in the towel if the dieter has a bad day or goes on a binge? Are your thoughts punctuated by imperatives (*always* or *never*)? Here are ways for you and the dieter to use your attitudes to work *for* you rather than against you.

Mind over Mouth

The first step in mastering your thoughts is to understand the human thinking process. One patient, Melissa, asked, "How can I change my thoughts when they just happen?" Most people agree with Melissa—that feelings are born from events. Let's take the case of Fred. If Fred's boss tells him he has done poorly on an assignment, Fred feels bad.

Event ⟶ Feeling

To apply this scheme to dieting, let's assume that Fred eats one half of an apple pie even though he has already reached his calorie level for the day. Fred feels guilty and is disgusted with himself. Instead of the one-way street this appeared to be, Fred is faced with a circular pattern of thinking. When he overeats, he feels bad. This makes him more prone to overeat. This leads to even worse feelings, and the circle goes on. Once Fred gets caught in this circular trap, it is difficult to escape.

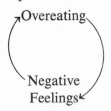

This is the way thinking occurs, right? WRONG!! Events do not cause feelings. Something intervenes between events and feelings. What is it?

$$\text{Event} \longrightarrow \ ? \longrightarrow \text{Feeling}$$

Our *reaction* to events determines how we feel. If we go back to Fred's traumas, we can see this clearly. When Fred's boss was upset with him, Fred felt bad because he said something to himself, something like, "I am failing, and it is embarrassing to have the boss angry with me." Fred could have avoided the bad feelings if his reaction had been different. He could have said to himself, "I usually do good work so this isn't so bad. Maybe the boss is having a bad day." You can see how two people could react very differently in the same situation, depending on their *self-statements*.

When Fred ate the apple pie, would his feelings have been different if he had the following self-statements?: "The pie has a lot of calories and I know I went over my limit for today. But I have done well the past four days and the best thing is to get back in line tomorrow." With this attitude, Fred isn't so likely to condemn himself and abandon the program. Here is the scheme that portrays the human thinking process:

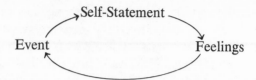

To avoid the circular trap of overeating and bad feelings, pay very close attention to your self-statements. This is true for both the dieter and the partner. We can now look at the five categories of thinking that are most important for your weight-loss program.

The Five Basic Areas of Thought

Dieters and partners have many thoughts about their eating behaviors. Some thoughts are helpful and some become mental quicksand (getting in is easier than getting out). These thoughts fall into five categories.

1. Light Bulb Thinking

Amy had been dieting for three weeks and had lost five pounds. During the third week she arrived for a coffee date with a neighbor and she was greeted by a freshly baked coffeecake. Amy couldn't resist having a piece with her coffee, and she enjoyed every bite. But when she got home, she felt so guilty about the cake that she decided she might as well give up and not even try.

My patients are often plagued with light bulb thinking; Amy is a good example. She had strict ideas about her diet, and coffeecake was not allowed. With light bulb thinking, she felt she was "off" the diet as soon as she ate some "illegal" food. Her thoughts (self-statements) were predictable: "What's the use? As soon as I get tempted, I give in. There's no point in dieting because I blow it every time."

This idea of being "on" or "off" a diet can be destructive. I want you to erase it from your mind and dispatch it to a faraway place. *All* foods are allowed on the Partnership Program; you can eat coffeecake and other foods as long as you watch the calories. As for the calories, suppose you are trying for 1200 each day. If you had 1201 calories one day, you certainly wouldn't have blown the diet. Would you condemn yourself for having 1210, or 1250, 1300, or 1400? These levels are probably far below your preprogram levels, so *any* reduction is an improvement. If you have 1500 calories one day, you are worse off than if you had taken in 1200 calories, but you are far better off than if you had consumed 3000 calories.

After a little practice Amy thought of new self-statements for the coffeecake situation: "Okay, I ate the cake. But I am in better control than ever before, and I really enjoyed the cake because I ate slowly. I know I am a little ahead of my calories since it is so early in the day, but I can be thrifty at lunch by having tuna salad and tomato instead of a sandwich."

Partner: You have to be on the lookout for light bulb thinking yourself. Remember that the dieter's behavior lies on a continuum that ranges from "perfect" to "terrible." There is much area between the two extremes, and any behavior should be judged in reference to how the dieter was doing before the program. One binge, or even a series of overeating episodes, does not mean the dieter is "off" the program. Cutting calories is a matter of give and take. Some days will be high and some will be low. On the "high" days it is important not to give up hope and for you to give the dieter all the support you can muster—so he or she will stick with the program.

2. *The Impossible Dream*

Your feelings about your weight and about a diet program will depend on your goals. Every day you compare your performance to the goals you have established for yourself. You know how good it feels to meet your goals, whether the goal was to clean the garage, to clear up old correspondence, to finish the shopping, or to eat just three cookies instead of the whole box.

If you set realistic goals, you will encounter happy feelings along the path to weight loss. If you set unrealistic goals, you doom yourself to feelings of inadequacy, disappointment, and guilt. Here are some examples of realistic and unrealistic goals. How would they affect you?

Situation	Impossible Goal	Realistic Goal
You are invited to a cocktail party.	"I won't drink anything but club soda. Unless they have raw vegetables, I won't eat anything."	"I'll have a tossed salad before I go so I won't be so hungry. I'll make one drink last as long as possible, and I'll have some food, but I'll stay away from the killers like potato chips, pretzels, and dips."
You're worried about the donuts you have every morning.	"No more donuts for me. I'll just have black coffee every morning from now on."	"This week I'll do without my usual donut on Tuesday and Thursday. If I have more donuts than I plan, I'll cut back at lunch."
You're helping a neighbor with a children's birthday party.	"There won't be anything there but cake and ice cream, so I just won't eat."	"I'll allow myself a small dish of ice cream and a piece of cake. Alice can serve the food and I'll organize the games so I won't have to spend much time around the tempting food."

The most impossible of the impossible dreams has to do with weight loss itself. Many dieters enter a program expecting to lose a great deal of weight. This is a healthy attitude, but not when miracles are expected immediately. Think how long it took to gain the weight you want to lose. It will take at least as long to lose it. Setting your sights on attainable goals will be the hallmark of success.

Here are some hints for goal setting:

a) *Think in the short term.* Concentrate on the weight loss you can achieve in the next week, not how you expect to look at the PTA ball in eleven months. When you lose a few pounds, you will feel proud, not discouraged because you still have such a long haul.

b) *Concentrate on behavior, not weight.* Your weight is a function of your eating behavior and your physical activity. The primary concern is *behavior,* so you should pat yourself on the back, not only for losing weight, but for following the program guidelines.

Partner: You can help with goal setting by not using the scale as your measure of success. If the dieter changes the way he or she eats, weight will decrease. The supportive strategies that appear at the end of each chapter can be used to reward behavior change as well as weight loss.

c) *Readjust your goals as needed.* The goals you set may be too difficult, or too easy. Renee started my program by saying that she would put her fork down between *every* bite. This wasn't a reasonable goal, so she decided to put her fork down 75 percent of the time. She also found this too difficult so she lowered her standard to 25 percent. She found this was too easy, so she made one more change—to 50 percent. She could accomplish this but she had to work hard to do it. As she became more proficient, she increased the goal gradually until now her goal is to put the fork down

80 percent of the time.

3. *The Awful Imperatives*

Many dieters get trapped by their choice of words. "Always" and "never" are imperatives that leave no room for error—or for leading a normal life.

Barbara entered my couples clinic with high hopes, but she got tangled in the imperative trap. She told herself, "I am never going to snack again." You can imagine how long she could live by this rule! When she did snack, she violated her "never" rule and felt miserable. These feelings made her more likely to surrender to the temptation of high-calorie foods.

After much group discussion Barbara banished the word "never" from her vocabulary. She recognized that snacking was an important part of her eating patterns and she was pleased that she could confine her snacks to scheduled times.

Examine your own thoughts. Have you told yourself that you will *never* eat chocolate cake, that you will *never* buy potato chips, that you will *always* order fish when you eat out, or that you will *always* jog a mile before you go to work? These are setups for disappointment.

Partner: Take the imperatives in your vocabulary and put them out to pasture. This applies to your standards as well as the standards you set for the dieter. You might have started this program with a burst of enthusiasm and with a resolution to be supportive *all* the time. Be as supportive as you can, but don't condemn yourself for being human and for failing to be perfect. Remember also that your expectations of the dieter are very important. How well your expectations are fulfilled will influence both you and the dieter. Be understanding when the dieter overeats, fails to follow the program guidelines, or doesn't lose weight. Your encouragement will have a positive effect in the long run.

4. *Dead-End Thinking*

Over the years, how many times have you said to yourself (perhaps unconsciously), "I was meant to be fat" or "I have absolutely no will power" or "I can't resist temptation"?

Partner, how often have you thought of the dieter and said, "There is no hope" or "He/she must have no will power at all" or "He/she will be fat forever"?

These dead-end thoughts can become troublesome for dieters and for their partners. If you have these thoughts repeatedly, there is a tendency to believe them. Your prophecies are then self-fulfilling. However, there is good news. Both of you can control these thoughts. The process we use to stop the thoughts is called, cleverly enough, thought stopping.

Every time you notice one of these dead-end thoughts racing through your mind, yell "STOP!" to yourself and imagine a red stop sign in your mind. Identify the destructive thought and rephrase it with a more rational response. Here are some examples:

Dieter's Statements

Original Statement	*Rational Restatement*
1. I have no will power.	1. I may have trouble in some situations, but I have better control than ever now that I am learning new habits.
2. I can't resist temptation.	2. I used to be much worse than I am now. In fact, I can resist temptation quite often.
3. I gained a pound this week. I will be fat forever.	3. I should concentrate on my new behaviors, not on the scale. My behav-

iors *are* changing, and the weight will follow.

4. This program won't work. I have failed on all the others.

4. I have never used such a systematic approach that focuses on social support. This program is different because it stresses new eating habits.

5. I'm stuck at home all day. It is impossible for me to lose.

5. Other people are stuck at home, and they lose weight. I have to use my new skills to master my own situation.

Partner's Statements

Original Statement

1. The dieter will be fat forever.

2. What can I do? This is the dieter's problem, not mine.

3. The dieter gained weight this week. There is no hope.

4. The dieter must not care about his/her appearance at all.

Rational Restatement

1. If we both change our habits, this program can really work.

2. I am not responsible for the problem, but I know I can help the dieter lose weight by doing the things I have learned in this program.

3. *Nobody* can lose weight every week. It is more important for me to be supportive because the dieter may be discouraged.

4. The dieter has been on dozens of diets, and I know it is not much fun. It must be hard to think about what you eat all the time.

| 5. The only way the dieter can lose is to cut out sweets. | 5. I know that sweets are hard to give up. The dieter can lose just by eating sweets in moderation. I can help by avoiding sweets myself when I am around the dieter. |

Before reading on, pinpoint your own thoughts and devise counterstatements. You should be able to mobilize the counterstatements on a moment's notice. When your mind launches a dead-end attack, deploy one of your anti–dead-end statements.

5. *Wishful Thinking*

Are you envious when you see slender people? Are you jealous that they don't have to watch what they eat? Is it disappointing that you have a weight problem while they are in control of their weight?

Nora was, until she had a frank discussion with her friend Kate. Nora said, "Kate, you are so lucky to be thin. You don't have half the worries I have." Kate was quick to say, "Of course I worry about what I eat. It is a constant struggle to keep thin. And besides, I have plenty of other problems that you are lucky you don't have."

Envying other people is simply a waste of time. It leads to discouragement and can make you detour from the road to reduction. If you catch yourself having wishful thoughts, scotch them right away!

Alternatives to Eating

Michelle has chocolate mint ice cream every afternoon. Why? Eating ice cream is the most attractive activity available. Suppose we offer Michelle the choice between the ice cream and a dream vacation to Hawaii? A new option is now available, and the ice cream would probably play second fiddle to the dream vacation. Michelle would have no trouble with ice cream if we could offer her similar enticements each day. Unfortunately, powerful attractions like dream vacations are not usually available, but this example does highlight an important point.

On many occasions, eating will occur unless another more rewarding option is available. If a person eats frequently, we can assume that eating is often the most rewarding option. This suggests a remedy for irresistible food urges —develop a repertoire of behaviors that are alternatives to eating. Many of my patients say, "I eat because I am bored." The obvious inference from this is—if you keep involved with alternative activities, you won't eat from boredom.

Partner, I'll bet your mind is spinning already from the ways you can think of to help the dieter with activities that are alternatives to eating. What does the dieter like to do? Can you help make these things happen at strategic times so that the dieter will be too involved to eat? Here is one clever ploy of Partnership Dieting in action. There will be more shortly.

One of my patients, Ed, had thirty-five pounds to lose. With Linda's help he was making fair progress in my clinic, but his weight really started falling when I introduced this system of alternative activities. Ed explained, "Since making love is one of our favorite activities, that's our first choice when I get those urges for cheese twists." Linda added, "Well, we *do* go jogging sometimes."

Dieter, fortify yourself with a list of enjoyable activities. Use this list at times when you feel the urge to eat. You and your partner can work well together in this area, but more about this in a moment. If possible, select behaviors that are incompatible with eating. Incompatible behaviors cannot occur simultaneously. For example, playing the tuba and jumping rope are incompatible behaviors—most people cannot do both at the same time. If somebody was possessed with uncontrollable urges to play the tuba, a regimen of rope jumping might just be the answer. Many activities are incompatible with eating. (If you are musically inclined, try eating and playing the harmonica at the same time!) I will give you hints about preparing your list of activities, but first read this case history.

Sandra has a high-pressure job in an employment agency. She is busy all day interviewing job hunters and telephoning personnel managers. Since she was occupied at work, she had no eating problems from nine to five. However, in the evenings and on weekends, snacking was her only means of relaxation, and she would succumb to eating urges like clockwork.

When I gave Sandra the assignment of finding other ways to relax, she admitted that she was taking the easy way out and indulging herself. She called her partner (her friend Ann) and developed a list of partner activities. Here is their list:

Play tennis	Play chess
See a movie	Frame some prints and
Browse in thrift shops	photographs
	Shop for new plants

Sandra made this list for solo activities:

Knit a sweater for her	Take a bubble bath
sister's baby	Look for new stationery
Practice the recorder	Call someone in the family
Go to the library	

Now when Sandra starts daydreaming about food, she immediately shifts gears and uses some activity from her list.

Planning Solo Activities

Some of your activities should be planned with your partner or with other people you enjoy. But you may not always have the luxury of being able to call on others when the urge to eat arises. Make a list of five activities you enjoy that are compatible with eating—or things that are so absorbing that you will forget about eating. When you are listing activities, use these guidelines:

1) Activities should be highly pleasurable. Weeding the garden may be satisfying and relaxing, but don't list it if you don't love it.

2) Exclude activities that involve food preparation. It is hard to forget food urges while you are preparing a tantalizing treat.

3) Choose diversions that occupy your hands. This will make them unavailable for transporting food from cupboard to mouth. Making pottery will serve this purpose; so will giving the dog a bath.

4) Exclude activities that require special equipment. Sculpting from a granite block is no good unless you work in a quarry. Hooking a rug is a good activity only if you are certain the canvas and the wool are in the house.

5) Add activities for the future. Have you always wanted to take guitar lessons, or have you wanted to learn to play the trombone? Does the idea of lifting weights intrigue you? Would you refinish the bedroom set if you had the time? Here is your chance to enrich your life and to derail your eating urges at the same time.

Planning Partnership Activities

Partner: Help plan the activities that you and the dieter can do together. Post the list in a conspicuous place, perhaps on the refrigerator door. When the urge strikes the dieter, suggest one of the activities on the list. Remember that the activities must be more enjoyable than eating. You and the dieter know which activities fit the bill. Use the guidelines listed above. If you think of wonderful activities, you both might wait on the edge of your chair for each and every eating urge!

Timing the Activities

If your eating urges are predictable and occur at reliable times, you can control them with time management. Change your schedule so you are busy when the urges hit. This will keep you away from food during prime time.

Toby scheduled meetings, returned phone calls, and did all her dictation in the mornings, so her afternoons were free for writing reports. She found from her Diet Diary that eating urges were most frequent in the afternoons. She shifted her schedule so her distracting work would occur in the afternoon. Her urges became less insistent and she had less trouble keeping her calories under control.

After his divorce, Alan's Saturdays were filled with new time-consuming chores—like going to the market, the Laundromat, and the dry cleaner. Because he was so bored and lonely, each activity was paired with a snack. His solution was to set his alarm half an hour earlier each morning. On Saturdays he did activities he enjoyed—visiting art galleries and museums. He also enrolled in a drawing class on Saturday mornings, and he is so busy that he sometimes forgets to eat lunch.

You remember from the section on the eating chain that eating can be controlled most effectively by interrupting the chain *before* you are confronted with food. It is important, therefore, to anticipate eating urges and to have your activities planned in advance. With you and your partner on the warpath, the urges won't stand a chance!

Supportive Strategies
1. Send a "thinking of you" card
2. Start a charm bracelet—with a tiny scale
3. Buy clothing one size too big so exchanging it will be flattering
4. Splurge on a very special dinner, but plan the meal in advance
5. Suggest dinner by candlelight

6. Buy a book on exotic love-making techniques
7. Plan a day at the nearest national park
8. Buy some fancy underwear
9. Window shop for an Oriental rug
10. Make a plant hanger for a favorite plant

CHAPTER 11

Day Seven–Physical Activity: Keeping Your Backfield in Motion

My patients think of exercise with a mixture of delight and dread. I recently asked one of my Partnership groups about their feelings on exercise. These were the first reactions:

Maggie: I used to love to play tennis and to ride bikes. But since I gained weight I get winded just thinking about exercising.

Dorothy: I have a solution. Whenever I get the urge to exercise, I lie down until it passes!

Heidi: Why all the talk about exercise? We are fat because we eat too much.

These patients weren't exactly ready to leap from their seats to do jumping jacks. But within three weeks, each of these women had significantly increased her physical activity—without pain, expense, or extra time. How? The answer in a moment. First, you and your partner answer the following questions to test your Exercise IQ.

	True	*False*
1. If I exercise, my appetite will increase so I will just eat more.	____	____
2. Exercise has to be strenuous for it to do any good.	____	____

3. I have to devote a lot of time to exercise, or the time is wasted.   _____   _____

Here is the good news: all three statements are false! This surprises many of my patients, especially those who think of exercise as a sweaty and grueling experience that makes you fit for nothing other than a body cast.

Partner: You can be instrumental in this part of the program. It is important for you to understand the role of exercise in a weight-loss program and to be aware of the type of physical activity that is best for the dieter. Armed with this, you and the dieter will learn dozens of ways to use more calories. Most of the activities are fun. For example, you can expend more calories by kissing than by gazing into someone's eyes!

Activity Can Curb Your Appetite

Martha echoed the sentiment of many dieters when she said, "If I went out and ran a mile before dinner, I'd come home and eat enough for three people." Martha's opinion changed when she came face-to-face with a few facts. Research has shown that exercise actually *decreases* appetite, especially in sedentary persons. Increasing your activity in modest amounts can help you lower your daily calorie levels. In fact, there are many benefits from regular exercise.

1) Your appetite will decrease and you will have a tendency to eat less.
2) You will expend more energy and will speed the rate of fat breakdown.
3) Your increased activity will make you feel better about yourself, and you will be more likely to stick with the program.
4) Your physical appearance will improve (beware of becoming irresistible!).
5) Your health will improve.

Activity Does NOT Have to Be Strenuous

Increasing your normal day-to-day activities can speed your weight loss. Let's say you decided to substitute one hour of walking each day for time you would normally be sitting. Your calorie expenditure would increase by 240 calories each day. This would amount to one pound's worth of calories every fifteen days, or twenty-four pounds in one year!

When you hear the word "exercise," what comes to mind—jogging, calisthenics, using an exercise bicycle? These *are* exercises, and good ones, too. But in the Partnership Program, exercise refers to *any* type of physical activity. This includes standing, walking, using stairs, and many other modes of movement that can boost your calorie expenditure. These "routine" activities are not strenuous and can be incorporated easily into your daily life.

Exercise Does NOT Have to Be Time-consuming

What discourages most people from exercising? "Too little time" ranks high on the list for most of my patients. It *does* take time to work out at the gym, to suit up at the pool, or to jog at the local park. But small amounts of exercise scattered throughout the day are just as helpful as a lengthy session of formal exercise. If you use the stairs at work five times each day and use 20 calories each time, the total expenditure of 100 calories is no different from the same 100 calories expended in a single session of wind sprints.

Dieters have even been known to *save* time by increasing physical activity. Climbing a flight of stairs is often faster than waiting for the elevator. Ruthie started walking six blocks to the train station instead of waiting for the bus. Usually she arrives before the bus.

Do I Overeat, or Do I Underexercise?

Sit down with your partner and give some thought to this question. Do you believe that exercise plays no part in your weight problem? Partner, do you think that the dieter's universe revolves around the refrigerator? Nearly everybody believes that excess weight results from excess eating. Consequently, most diet programs pay little attention to exercise. Several startling facts point to the importance of physical activity for the dieter.

Since 1900 the percentage of obese people in the American population has doubled. "Of course," my patients say, "food is much more available now and we eat much more." WRONG! The average American consumes 10 percent *fewer* calories today than in 1900. Why the increase in obesity? Physical inactivity is one major reason.

Normal living requires less and less physical activity because of increased use of energy-saving devices. The most obvious of these devices is the automobile. Imagine how much energy you would expend if you traveled everywhere by foot. Elevators and escalators are other good examples, and there are many more. There are devices to open your garage door, brush your teeth, dry your hair, process your food, carve your turkey, wash your dishes, compact your garbage, mow your lawn, saw your wood, roll down your car windows, crush your ice, turn off your TV from afar, and so on. The energy expense for any of these tasks is small, but the cumulative effect of all the activities is immense.

Notice that the changes in physical activity have not been in jogging, swimming, calisthenics, or other rigorous activities. Rather, the change has occurred in our normal day-to-day routine of going to work, washing clothes, preparing meals, and so forth. This explains why you and your partner will be learning how to increase the energy expenditure in your daily activities. This approach to exercise is easy, enjoyable, and beneficial.

Exercise—Your Heart versus Your Waist

I recently conducted an exercise program for the employees of a large corporation in Philadelphia. Some people joined to improve their health; others joined to improve their figure (lose weight). Different types of activity are useful for each purpose. We will concentrate on activities for weight loss, but it is also important to consider the relationship between exercise and your health.

Regular exercise is associated with reduced risk of coronary heart disease (the number one killer in America). People who exercise regularly have fewer heart attacks and strokes than sedentary people. If active people do have heart attacks, they are more likely to recover. You can improve nearly every circulatory function in your body with proper exercise.

The cardiovascular effect of exercise depends on the type of activity, its difficulty, its duration, and its frequency. Aerobic activities (running, swimming, cycling, rope jumping, etc.) are preferable to anaerobic activities (lifting weights, isometrics, shoveling snow, etc.). Aerobic activities produce a sustained increase in oxygen use and promote increased cardiac efficiency. Anaerobic activities increase muscle strength but do little for your heart.

Your heart is like any other muscle; it must be exercised regularly to stay in top condition. To improve your cardiovascular functioning, you must exercise at least three times each week. During each session, your heart rate (pulse) must be at least at 75 percent of maximum for at least twenty minutes. (You can measure your pulse with your fingertips, at your wrist or your neck. Count the number of beats in fifteen seconds, then multiply by four to find the number of beats per minute.) Your maximum heart rate depends on your age and several other factors. You can estimate your maximum heart rate by subtracting your age from 220. For example, if you are forty years old,

$$220 - 40 \text{ (age)} = 180 \text{ beats per minute}$$
$$\text{(maximum heart rate)}$$

To give your body a good workout, you must increase your heart rate to 75 percent of the maximum of 180 beats per minute (135 beats per minute). If you are thirty years old, the figures are:

$$220 - 40 \text{ (age)} = 180 \text{ beats per minute}$$
$$(75\% = 143 \text{ beats per minute})$$

Following these guidelines, a typical exercise session might consist of warm-up exercises for ten minutes, slow jogging for five minutes, fast running for twenty minutes, then slow jogging again for five minutes. I wholeheartedly support this type of exercise. It is one of the few positive behaviors you can perform to reduce your risk for heart disease. I realize, however, that this type of exercise is not possible or realistic for many people. If you do not have the motivation, stamina, or time for such a program, you are in the majority. At some point you may be able to work your way up to a strenuous regimen, but in the meantime there are many easier ways to exercise.

Unless you are in excellent condition, you should not try a strenuous exercise program without first consulting your physician. When sedentary people stress their bodies, they usually suffer little other than sore muscles and aching joints. But some people pay a much dearer price. Your physician is in the best position to know how much, how hard, and how often you should exercise.

Exercising for your waistline does not require strenuous activity. You can use 200 calories preparing for a marathon or strolling through the park with your partner. As you read about the ways of increasing your activity, keep one thing in mind. Select activities that are fun! Do something that you would like to do again and again. Unpleasant activities will not be repeated, so do your best to have fun!

Energizing Your Routine

You are about to be activated! The best way to increase your physical activity is to make small changes in your daily routine. *Everyone* can make these changes, and best of all, these changes are likely to become lifetime habits. You can live with the changes I will suggest. This makes you a good candidate for permanent weight loss.

Routine exercise:

Doesn't	*Does*
Hurt	Burn calories
Take time	Help your self-concept
Require equipment	Improve your health
Cost anything	Let your partner help
Make you perspire	
Make you sore	

I will suggest many ways for you to become more active. They are all based on one principle: *use every opportunity to expend more energy.* When you and your partner discuss these methods, you will undoubtedly think of methods that fit *your* routine. Here are ways to burn up more calories every day without changing your life.

Use Stairs Whenever Possible

Climbing stairs uses more calories per minute than calisthenics, swimming, bicycling—even jogging. This is a powerful way to shed pounds because of the frequent opportunity to use stairs. However, most people don't think of using the stairs as a way to increase exercise. Some of my own research has shown this clearly.

With two colleagues, I recently conducted a study to

measure stair usage in public places. We sent observers to three public locations where stairs and escalators were side by side: a shopping mall, a train station, and a bus terminal. More than 45,000 people were observed making this choice between stairs and escalators. Only 5 percent chose the stairs even though the stair users usually arrived at the top more quickly. Of the overweight people, only 1 percent used the stairs!

We then put up a sign that encouraged people to use the stairs. The sign tripled the number of people using the stairs and produced a six-fold increase in the number of overweight people on the stairs. This shows how easy it is to make such a change in activity. Here are some methods to increase your stair use.

1. *Use the stairs when shopping.* The next time you are in a building with adjacent stairs and escalators, conduct your own study of whether people use the stairs. Then, be one of the few who are clever enough to use the stairs. In some public buildings, particularly department stores, you may have to search for the stairs. The effort will pay off.

2. *Use the stairs at work.* If your job demands that you move between floors of a building, you have a golden opportunity to increase your activity level. Use the stairs rather than an elevator or escalator. Remember to do only as much as you can without being uncomfortable, then gradually increase the number of stairs you climb. For example, if you make eight trips to another floor on an average day, start out by making two of the trips via the stairs. If this is easy, go to three, then four . . . The same applies when you arrive at work. If you work on the tenth floor, take the elevator to the eighth floor, then walk the remaining two flights. Increase the walking as your fitness improves.

If you don't have the occasion to move between floors, there are several ways to create the occasion. Messages that might ordinarily be delivered over the telephone can be delivered in person. Also, make it a point to use the rest room on another floor.

3. *Use the stairs at home.* Having stairs in your home is a real plus. The stairs can become an exercise machine—at no cost. Rather than allowing items to collect before taking them to another floor, make several trips. If you ask other members of the household to bring things to you (your coat, a pencil, etc.), start being your own courier. One patient, Ann, was very resourceful with the stairs in her house. "We have a bathroom on the first floor and one on the second floor. I always go to the bathroom on the floor I am not on." Each time you follow Ann's lead and use the stairs, you will be using calories at a rapid rate.

Partner: When you are with the dieter in public places, seek out the stairs. You could be the scout who finds exactly where the stairs are (you have an important mission). In most public places like airports, hotels, and shopping malls, stairs are easy to find. Set a good example by using the stairs whenever you are with the dieter. If you and the dieter are co-workers, use the stairs together whenever possible. You may want to get your coffee on a different floor, or have the dieter visit you frequently if you work on different floors.

Ways to Increase Your Walking

Your legs can be your best friends! Walking is one of the best activities for weight loss. It is something we do routinely, and it is not difficult to increase the amount we do. It is an efficient means of burning calories—walking a mile uses essentially the same energy as running a mile. Because walking is easy, is not painful, and can be fun, it has the potential to become a long-term activity for you. There are many ways to increase your walking. Here are a few that my patients find most helpful.

1. *Park some distance from your destination.* Shoppers are known for circling the aisles of cars in search of a parking spot near the door. You can increase your walking by parking several hundred feet from the entrance of the store. Not only will you increase your exercise, but you will avoid the frustration of seeing another shopper pull into a choice

spot, and you may arrive at the store sooner because you won't devote time to finding the perfect parking spot.

If you are driving to a friend's house, park several blocks away. The same principle holds for a trip downtown. Intentionally park several blocks from your destination. You will feel better and will lose weight faster.

2. *Get on and off the bus before your stop.* Short of blizzards and cloudbursts, get off one stop before your destination. If the traffic is heavy, you may arrive before the bus. Do the same at the beginning of the trip by walking to the next bus stop before getting on.

3. *Abandon short-cuts.* Use any opportunity to increase your walking, even if it means forgetting some of your favorite short-cuts. Whether it is through a neighbor's yard, a parking lot, or a park, take the long way around.

4. *When you want a nap, take a walk.* Research has shown that exercise provides an increase in energy level that can last for as much as four to six hours. If you feel weary, take a walk. The scenery might cheer you up, and the activity will pick you up. Also, walking uses more calories than lying down.

5. *Walk at work.* When you want a drink of water, use the cooler at the farthest point, not the nearest. If you need to mail a letter, find a distant mail chute. Use a rest room on another floor, and use the stairs. Any form of movement will help.

More Methods for Movement

My patients have devised many innovative ways for increasing exercise. Here are some that may help you and your partner:

1. Use fewer wastebaskets at home. You will then have to walk more to throw things away, and the baskets will require emptying more often. This will be especially good if you have "trash duty."

2. Form an office partnership or club to seek out restaurants farther from the office. The walk will provide a pleasant chance to visit, and you will broaden your spectrum of lunch spots.

3. When you are on the phone, stand rather than sit. Standing requires more calories than sitting, so turning your phone into a "walkie-talkie" can help with your weight.

4. Are there sounds that prompt you to eat—perhaps the coffee wagon bell or the music of the ice cream truck? These signals can be as alluring to the dieter as the sirens' songs were to Ulysses. Instead of stuffing your ears with wax, use the sound as a signal to walk. Take a quick trip up and down the stairs, or go out for a stroll.

5. Don't use the remote control on your TV.

6. Don't stack dishes on a tray when you clear the table. Remove them one at a time.

7. Store things far from where you need them. The laundry detergent, for example, can be stored in the pantry so you have an extra trip each time the clothes get dirty.

Partner: You have probably thought of even more ways for you and the dieter to increase activity. Discuss these methods with the dieter and see which ones fit comfortably into your daily routines. Remember that the new activities must be enjoyable or they will not be maintained. The pleasure factor will be greatest if you take part in the activities with the dieter and if you encourage the dieter at every opportunity.

You can help increase the dieter's activity by taking the lead whenever possible. When you are driving, park some distance from the destination. Get up to disembark from the bus one or more stops early. Move to the stairs whenever you have the opportunity to climb instead of ride.

Supportive Strategies

Many supportive strategies can be used to encourage increased physical activity. Here are some ways both of you can do nice things for each other and increase the calories you burn at the same time:

1. Go for a romantic walk
2. Get bicycles so you can sightsee together
3. Get a jump rope for the office, to use for a few minutes at free times
4. Go bowling
5. Walk around some nice part of your city where you haven't been lately
6. Give your partner a book of IOUs for ten hours of jogging, tennis, racquetball, etc.
7. Buy a pedometer to check the miles your partner walks and runs
8. Make a date for some physical affection
9. Have a contest to see who can climb the most stairs in a week. The loser pays for the next movie you see.
10. Learn a game you have never played (squash, tennis, etc.)

Calorie Values of Various Exercises

Increasing your physical activity will be easier if you know the number of calories you will burn for various activities. Do you know, for example, whether you expend more calories washing the floor or weeding the garden, playing tennis or jogging, standing or using a typewriter? I have prepared the following chart to answer all your questions about calories and exercise.

The number of calories you burn depends on the activity and on your body weight (the more you weigh, the more energy it takes to perform a task). The chart includes values for different body weights. The calorie values represent the number of calories you expend doing ten minutes of *continuous* activity.

CALORIES EXPENDED FOR 10 MINUTES OF ACTIVITY

Activity	Body Weight				
	125 Pounds	150 Pounds	175 Pounds	200 Pounds	250 Pounds
Personal Necessities					
Sleeping	10	12	14	16	20
Sitting (Reading or Watching TV)	10	12	14	16	18
Sitting (Talking)	15	18	21	24	30
Dressing or Washing	26	32	37	42	53
Standing	12	14	16	19	24
Locomotion					
Walking Downstairs	56	67	78	88	111
Walking Upstairs	146	175	202	229	288
Walking—2 mph	29	35	40	46	58
Walking—4 mph	52	62	72	81	102
Running—5.5 mph	90	108	125	142	178
Running—7 mph	118	141	164	187	232
Running—12 mph (Sprint)	164	197	228	258	326
Cycling—5.5 mph	42	50	58	67	83
Cycling—13 mph	89	107	124	142	178
Housework					
Making Beds	32	39	46	52	65
Washing Floors	38	46	53	60	75

| | Body Weight | | | | |
Activity	125 Pounds	150 Pounds	175 Pounds	200 Pounds	250 Pounds
Washing Windows	35	42	48	54	69
Dusting	22	27	31	35	44
Preparing a Meal (without Snitching)	32	39	46	52	65
Shoveling Snow	65	78	89	100	130
Light Gardening	30	36	42	47	59
Weeding Garden	49	59	68	78	98
Mowing Grass (Power)	34	41	47	53	67
Mowing Grass (Manual)	38	45	52	58	74
Sedentary Occupation					
Sitting Writing	15	18	21	24	30
Light Office Work	25	30	34	39	50
Standing (Light Activity)	20	24	28	32	40
Typing 40 Words/Min (Electric)	19	23	27	31	39
Light Work					
Assembly Work in Factory	20	24	28	32	40
Auto Repair	35	42	48	54	69
Carpentry	32	38	44	51	64
Bricklaying	28	34	40	45	57
Farming Chores	32	38	44	51	64
House Painting	29	35	40	46	58

Heavy Work					
Pick-and-Shovel Work	56	67	78	88	110
Chopping Wood	60	73	84	96	121
Dragging Logs	158	189	220	252	315
Drilling Coal	79	95	111	127	159
Recreation					
Badminton or Volleyball	43	52	65	75	94
Baseball (except Pitcher)	39	47	54	62	78
Basketball	58	70	82	93	117
Bowling (Nonstop)	56	67	78	90	111
Canoeing—4 mph	90	109	128	146	182
Dancing (Moderate)	35	42	48	55	69
Dancing (Vigorous)	48	57	66	75	94
Football	69	83	96	110	137
Golfing	33	40	48	55	68
Horseback Riding	56	67	78	90	112
Ping-Pong	32	38	45	52	64
Racquetball/Squash	75	90	104	117	144
Skiing (Alpine)	80	96	112	128	160
Skiing (Water)	60	73	88	104	130
Skiing (Cross-Country)	98	117	138	158	194
Swimming (Backstroke—20 Yd/Min)	32	38	45	52	64
Swimming (Crawl—20 Yd/Min)	40	48	56	63	80
Tennis	56	67	80	92	115

CHAPTER 12

Your Timetable for Success: The Sixteen-Week Partnership Diet Schedule

Now you and your partner begin the most intriguing (and important) part of the program—the sixteen-week schedule for using the Partnership Diet plan. *You* will be in command of your weight. You will apply the principles you have learned in order to structure a program that is specific to *your* eating patterns. The upcoming weeks will teach you more about weight control than most dieters learn in a lifetime.

Why a sixteen-week schedule? In the past seven days you and your partner have learned the principles of Partnership Dieting and have practiced some of the techniques that will make you a weight-control expert. This is adequate time to acquaint yourself with the program, but is not enough time to reach your goal weight, or to make permanent changes in your eating habits. In my clinics I use a sixteen-week schedule for implementing the program. This allows time to practice each of the techniques and to mold the program into each patient's lifestyle. This chapter includes the sixteen-week schedule with a step-by-step guide for you and your partner to speed down the path to lasting weight loss.

At this point your thoughts may be like Vicki's: "My

head is buzzing with behaviors, attitudes, and activities. What do I do first?" The unruly conglomeration of thoughts in your mind will soon become an orderly system for weight reduction. For the next sixteen weeks you and your partner will be experimenting with new techniques. You are about to see how powerful Partnership Dieting can be!

The remaining chapters in this book will be invaluable as you progress through the next sixteen weeks. Chapters 13 and 14 contain crisis intervention techniques for the two most common diet crises: special events where eating is the *main* event, and the disheartening halt to weight loss that nearly every dieter experiences. Chapter 15 will answer your most pressing questions about dieting, nutrition, and exercise. (Take the Weight-Loss Wisdom Test with your partner to see who knows most about dieting.) In Chapters 16 and 17 you will use Magic Recipes for scrumptious low-calorie dishes, and you will have a month's worth of menus for delicious eating (the menus include fast foods and frozen convenience foods, along with calorie values for dozens of meals). Chapter 18 will describe how to take control of your weight forever, and will give you "The Last Word" on dieting.

Partner, here is where you and the dieter implement the new techniques you have learned. For each of the sixteen weeks, you will have a set of behaviors that corresponds to the dieter's behaviors. The dieter's weight loss will be greater, easier, and will be maintained longer if you are conscientious about your role in the program. You are *not* a spectator. Your active participation will boost the dieter's weight loss and will make for a creative working relationship. You will have important responsibilities in the program, but the rewards will be great. The dieting process is like a bicycle built for two. When *both* people do the peddling, you reach your destination faster and with a cooperative spirit that pleases everyone.

Dieter *and* partner, you are both making important

changes. Depending on your individual lifestyles, these changes may not be easy. The support you give each other can be one of the most important factors in the diet. Partner, you know how difficult it is for the dieter to lose weight and to keep it off. Maladaptive eating habits that have occurred for years cannot be changed overnight. However, changes *can* be made, and your support and encouragement can speed the process along.

Dieter, your partner is to be saluted for helping you with the program. Few people are willing and able to be good partners in a diet program. Your partner's task is not easy. In some cases the partner's changes will be as difficult as yours.

The moral? Both of you need support during the program. It is easy to take the other's behavior for granted, but remember that he or she will respond positively if you acknowledge important accomplishments. Provide as much emotional support as possible. There are seventy specific supportive strategies in Chapters 5 through 11. Use these to reward each other for stunning performances, or even for minor adjustments. Think of your own supportive strategies, and use them freely.

Measuring Your Progress

The techniques you will be using are drawn from the last seven chapters, so be certain to reread the chapters before practicing the procedures. Some of the behaviors will not be appropriate for you (for example, shopping from a list if you do not do the food shopping). Use the behaviors that apply to your lifestyle, but do not rule out a behavior because it is too hard or because it feels awkward. These may be the behaviors you need most. They will get easier as times goes on.

There are two critical record-keeping procedures to use throughout the entire program—the Diet Diary, and the Daily Log.

The Diet Diary

The Diet Diary (see Chapters 5 and 6) is to be used *every* day. The diary is your weight repellent. It gives you an instant record of your calorie intake and allows you to track your progress from day to day. My patients are almost unanimous in their claim that filling out the Diet Diary is the single most important technique in the program. Make copies of the diary page in Chapter 5 and keep the diary with you at all times. Fill it out immediately after (or before) you eat. Discuss the results with your partner. Together you will use this information for each stage of the program.

The Daily Log

Your goal is to lose weight by making permanent changes in your eating, attitudes, and activity. You can identify strengths and weaknesses in your program only by measuring your dieting behaviors. The Daily Log will accomplish this.

The Daily Log is a simple form on which you record the Partnership techniques. You will have a new Daily Log each week. Each log will list the behaviors you will be using for that week, so you will have a record of *how* you are eating.

Partner, your behavior is as important as the dieter's. The Partnership Program includes a Daily Log for you, so you and the dieter will be able to review the accomplishments you are making. More about your log shortly. Read the next section for a description of how the log is completed.

As an example, I have included a Daily Log from one of my patients, Beth (see Figure 1). This log is from week seven of the program; Beth was practicing six behaviors that week. At the end of each day Beth recorded points for each behavior. She awarded points according to how well she used the techniques. The scoring system allows 5 points for doing a behavior all of the time, 3 points for most of the time, 1 point for some of the time, and 0 points for not at all. You also award yourself points for your calorie total, depending on how close to your goal you are. You can add the points to get a total for each day and then add your daily totals to get a total for the week.

The point system has several purposes. First, you compare your weekly total to the maximum points for the week. Second, the point system allows you to reward yourself for making small and gradual changes in your eating habits. Notice that you get points even when your behavior is not "perfect" and when your calorie total is somewhat over your goal for the day. I structure the Daily Logs this way to underscore the fact that you are not "on" or "off" the diet. You should not consider yourself either "perfect" or "bad." Any progress is useful.

Let's examine Beth's record. On Monday she awarded herself 5 points for each behavior, except for removing the serving dishes, and for using smaller utensils (and she did these *most* of the time). She had 1132 calories for the day, so she earned 5 points in that category. Her total of 31 points for Monday was excellent. On Tuesday she failed to use three of the behaviors at all (thus her three 0s). On another diet Beth would have felt miserable because she didn't use the prescribed behaviors. With the Partnership Program, Beth said to herself, "I could have done better, but I still got 5 points for filling out the diary, and my calorie total of 1653 got me one point. This shows I did *something*."

After carefully reviewing her own record, Beth discovered that her highest calorie days were the days when she was inconsistent with the behaviors. She could then make the necessary changes. When she added her points for the week, she found that her total of 194 was fairly close to the maximum score of 245 (she had 79 percent of the maximum score).

DIETER'S DAILY LOG – WEEK ___7___

POINTS: ALL OF THE TIME = 5 POINTS
          MOST OF THE TIME = 3 POINTS
          SOME OF THE TIME = 1 POINT
          NOT AT ALL   = 0 POINTS

Beth
NAME

	DAY						
	Mon.	Tues.	Wed.	Thurs.	Fri.	Sat.	Sun.
1. DID I FILL OUT THE DIET DIARY AFTER EATING?	5	5	3	5	3	5	5
2. *Did I keep food out of sight?*	5	3	3	1	1	5	3
3. *Did I avoid being a food dispenser?*	5	5	5	5	5	5	5
4. *Did I remove serving dishes after serving?*	3	0	5	5	5	3	5
5. *Did I use smaller utensils?*	3	0	5	5	5	3	5
6. *Did I leave the table after eating?*	5	0	5	5	5	3	5
HOW MANY CALORIES DID I HAVE TODAY? **FOR WOMEN** 1000-1200 = 5 POINTS 1200-1500 = 3 POINTS 1500-1700 = 1 POINT ABOVE 1700 = 0 POINTS **FOR MEN** 1200-1500 = 5 POINTS 1500-1800 = 3 POINTS 1800-2000 = 1 POINT ABOVE 2000 = 0 POINTS	5 (1132)	1 (1653)	3 (1370)	5 (1080)	5 (1103)	3 (1446)	5 (1161)
TOTAL POINTS FOR THE DAY	31	14	29	31	29	27	33

TOTAL POINTS FOR THIS WEEK: ___194___

MAXIMUM POINTS FOR THIS WEEK: ___245___

Each week calculate your total score and then divide by the maximum score to determine your percentage of maximum. For example, if the maximum score for one week is 206 points, and you score 158 points, your percentage is $\frac{158}{206} = 77\%$. These are the guidelines to use for your percentages each week.

% of Maximum Score	Rating
88%–100%	Outstanding
75%– 87%	Excellent
60%– 74%	Very Good
45%– 59%	Good
30%– 44%	Adequate
0%– 29%	Poor

The Partner's Daily Log

Partner, your Daily Log is similar to the dieter's. For each week of the program, you will be using the special techniques described in the earlier chapters. Your techniques will complement the dieter's techniques, and your mutual effort will solve even the most persistent problems. Your log is scored just as the dieter's log is scored.

Why the Daily Log for you? First, you deserve credit for the changes *you* make. The Daily Log is the best method for documenting and measuring these changes. You and the dieter can observe your log and note the progress you are making. Second, you will have a clear picture of the behaviors that are most strongly related to the dieter's weight loss. Third, the Daily Log reminds you that constant vigilance is necessary and that your behaviors are important to the dieter's success. Fourth, the score from your log will provide reinforcement during difficult times because you will be able to feel proud of your accomplishments.

Here is a sample Partner's Daily Log, filled out by

Steve, Beth's partner (see Figure 2). Steve's behaviors were to be used in conjunction with Beth's behaviors. If Beth was to avoid being a food dispenser, Steve was to avoid offering food to Beth. Steve was able to look over his scores to see which techniques were most helpful to Beth. Steve could compare his score to the maximum score, to evaluate *his* behavior change. He earned 179 of a possible 210 points. The 85 percent of maximum score showed that his work was "excellent."

Taking Command

For each of the next sixteen weeks, I will list the techniques that you and your partner will be practicing. There will be different techniques for each week. The techniques are to be listed in your Daily Log for each week. I have provided a blank Daily Log for the dieter (Figure 3) and a blank Daily Log for the partner (Figure 4). Make sixteen copies of each log, one for each week. The logs I have provided are blank so you can fill in the behaviors that are to be used for any given week. For example, in week five there are two behaviors for the dieter—eating all food in the same place, and eating meals and snacks at scheduled times. During week five the dieter should list these two techniques in one of the blank Daily Logs, then use the completed log for the entire week. The partner should do the same for each of the sixteen weeks.

For the dieter, there are two items that appear in *every* Daily Log. The first—"Did I fill out the Diet Diary?" This behavior is so important that you need to keep a record of it each and every week. The second item is your calorie level. Use your Diet Diary each day to total your calories. Then enter the number into your Daily Log and award yourself the appropriate number of points. These two items are already entered into the blank Daily Log.

PARTNER'S DAILY LOG – WEEK __7__

(BEHAVIORS WHEN WITH DIETER)　　　NAME _Steve_

POINTS:　ALL OF THE TIME　= 5 POINTS
　　　　　MOST OF THE TIME　= 3 POINTS
　　　　　SOME OF THE TIME　= 1 POINT
　　　　　NOT AT ALL　　　　= 0 POINTS

	DAY						
	Mon.	Tues.	Wed.	Thur.	Fri.	Sat.	Sun.
1. DID I DISCUSS THE DIET DIARY WITH THE DIETER?	5	5	5	5	5	5	5
2. Did I keep food out of sight?	5	3	3	3	5	5	3
3. Did I avoid offering food to the dieter?	5	5	5	3	5	5	5
4. Were serving dishes removed from the table?	3	3	5	1	5	3	5
5. Did I use smaller utensils?	3	5	5	3	5	5	5
6. Did I leave the table after eating?	5	0	5	5	5	3	5
TOTAL POINTS FOR DAY	26	21	28	20	30	26	28

TOTAL POINTS FOR THIS WEEK: _179_

MAXIMUM POINTS FOR THIS WEEK: _210_

DIETER'S DAILY LOG –WEEK_____

NAME _____

POINTS: ALL OF THE TIME   = 5 POINTS
       MOST OF THE TIME = 3 POINTS
       SOME OF THE TIME = 1 POINT
       NOT AT ALL   = 0 POINTS

	DAY						
1. DID I FILL OUT THE DIET DIARY AFTER EATING ?							

HOW MANY CALORIES DID I HAVE TODAY ?
 	
FOR WOMEN
  1000–1200 = 5 POINTS
  1200–1500 = 3 POINTS
  1500–1700 = 1 POINT
  ABOVE 1700 = 0 POINTS
 	
FOR MEN
  1200–1500 = 5 POINTS
  1500–1800 = 3 POINTS
  1800–2000 = 1 POINT
  ABOVE 2000 = 0 POINTS							

TOTAL POINTS FOR DAY							

TOTAL POINTS FOR THIS WEEK _____
MAXIMUM POINTS FOR THIS WEEK _____

PARTNER'S DAILY LOG – WEEK＿＿＿＿

(BEHAVIORS WHEN WITH DIETER)   NAME＿＿＿＿

POINTS: ALL OF THE TIME   = 5 POINTS
         MOST OF THE TIME   = 3 POINTS
         SOME OF THE TIME   = 1 POINT
         NOT AT ALL   = 0 POINTS

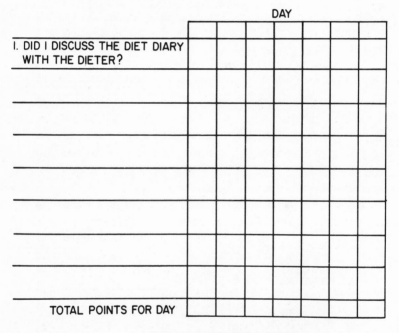

DAY

I. DID I DISCUSS THE DIET DIARY WITH THE DIETER?

TOTAL POINTS FOR DAY

TOTAL POINTS FOR THIS WEEK:＿＿＿＿＿

MAXIMUM POINTS FOR THIS WEEK:＿＿＿＿＿

Partner, there is one behavior that is already entered into your blank Daily Log: "Did I discuss the Diet Diary with the dieter?" This technique is very effective and should become routine. By recording your discussion each day, you will remind the dieter to follow through with the diary and you will be able to offer the support the dieter needs.

Each week's material also includes a record of the Weekly Weigh-In. This includes a record of the dieter's weight and the partner's weight. Dieters are sometimes reluctant to reveal their weight to their partner ("What they don't know can't hurt them!"). This happens frequently with husband-wife partnerships. After much discussion I usually convince my patients that partners will not lapse into a coma from the shock of discovering the dieter's weight. After the initial embarrassment there is little problem in subsequent weeks.

If the partner is dieting, the partner's weight should be recorded each week. Even if the partner is not trying to lose weight, a weekly weigh-in with the dieter can be helpful. This makes the weigh-in a special event and shows the dieter how committed the partner is.

Remember to read over the material from Chapters 5 through 11 when you are implementing the techniques. There is a tendency to disregard some of the behaviors and to use other behaviors before they are prescribed. It is best to use the techniques in the prearranged order and to give your best effort to each behavior. Toward the end of the program you will select the behaviors that are most helpful for *you,* but in order to make an educated decision, you must give each of the techniques a fair shake.

You may be wondering what will happen after the sixteen weeks. Rest assured that I will discuss the maintenance of your weight loss and methods for losing even more weight. The months and years that follow are as important as the weeks you devote to starting the program. Once you master the Partnership Program, you can come back to this book at any point in your life and shed any pounds you may gain.

Let's Go!

Week One

The very first item of business is to fill out the Diet Diary. Read the discussion of the Diet Diary in Chapter 5, and be sure to look up the calories of your foods in the appendixes. Look over the diary each day with your partner to identify problem foods. Remember to fill out the diary *immediately* after eating—or before, if you prefer to prerecord.

Second, keep your calories to 1200 (for women) or 1500 (for men). This item and the Diet Diary technique are already listed on your blank Daily Log. Therefore, the blank Daily Log can be used just as it is for week one.

Partner, your first behavior is to discuss the Diet Diary with the dieter. Since this technique is already listed on your Daily Log, you can use it as it is for week one. Fill out the Daily Log at the end of each day, and total your points.

Techniques for the Daily Log

Dieter's Techniques
1. Fill out the Diet Diary immediately after eating (or before, if you prefer to prerecord).
2. Limit calories to 1200 (women) or 1500 (men).

Partner's Techniques
1. Discuss the Diet Diary with the dieter.

Weekly Weigh-In
Dieter's Weight _____   Date _____
Partner's Weight _____

Week Two

Completing the Diet Diary is a new and unusual task for many dieters. Filling out the diary will become second nature before long, and it will take only seconds to record all the valuable information. In the meantime I want you to practice with the diary for another week without the addition of other new techniques, just to make sure it becomes an automatic response.

What have you and your partner discovered from the Diet Diary? Are there certain foods that appear often? Do you tend to eat most of your food during certain meals? These are the questions to bear in mind as you ponder the results of the diary.

Techniques for the Daily Log

Dieter's Techniques
1. Fill out the Diet Diary immediately after eating (or before, if you prefer to prerecord).
2. Limit calories to 1200 (women) or 1500 (men).

Partner's Techniques
1. Discuss the Diet Diary with the dieter.

Weekly Weigh-In
Dieter's Weight _____   Date _____
Partner's Weight _____

Week Three

This is the week for the Extended Diet Diary. The discussion of this technique is in Chapter 6. Copy the Extended Diary in Chapter 6, and fill it out each day this week. You will be recording the times, places, people, feelings, and activities that accompany eating. You and your partner will form a diagnostic impression of your eating patterns with this new knowledge.

As you and your partner begin to see patterns emerge, think ahead for ways to combat the problems that contribute to weight gain. Are you aware of the times you eat, the activities you do while you eat (TV?) . . . ?

Techniques for the Daily Log

Dieter's Techniques

1. Fill out the Extended Diet Diary immediately before or after eating.
2. Limit calories to 1200 (women) or 1500 (men).

Partner's Techniques

1. Discuss the Extended Diet Diary with the dieter.

Weekly Weigh-In

Dieter's Weight _____   Date _____

Partner's Weight _____

Week Four

In Chapter 3 you learned about protecting your eating environment. From your Extended Diet Diary you will know the people, places, activities, and so forth that are associated with eating. The techniques for this week will help you separate eating from these factors. This will help minimize the number of environmental cues that provoke eating.

The first protection techniques deal with the sight of food and associated activities. The first behavior, leaving some food on your plate, will help break the age-old habit of eating everything you are served. Being at the mercy of the server is not good for a dieter. The second behavior, doing nothing else while eating, will help make eating a pure activity—you won't be distracted by other things. This will help you enjoy food more.

Techniques for the Daily Log

Dieter's Techniques

1. Fill out the Diet Diary immediately before or after eating.
2. Leave some food on your plate at each meal.
3. Do nothing else while eating.
4. Limit calories to 1200 (women) or 1500 (men).

Partner's Techniques
1. Discuss the Diet Diary with the dieter.
2. Leave some food on your plate when with the dieter.
3. Do nothing else while eating with the dieter.

Weekly Weigh-In
> Dieter's Weight _____   Date _____
> Partner's Weight _____

Week Five

Week five will find you using several more techniques to keep activities, times, and places separate from eating. Many dieters know that places can provoke eating. For some it is the bed, for others it is the easy chair by the TV, and for others it is the car. These associations can be broken with a simple procedure—eat all food in the same place. The time of day can also be a sure-fire trigger for eating. Time can work in your favor if you eat only at scheduled eating times. Snacks are legal on the Partnership Program—as long as you schedule them.

Partners can be important helpers by limiting the times and places they eat while they are with the dieter. Reread Chapter 7 for some useful methods of accomplishing this.

Techniques for the Daily Log

Dieter's Techniques
1. Fill out the Diet Diary immediately before or after eating.
2. Eat all food in the same place.
3. Eat all meals and snacks at scheduled times.
4. Limit calories to 1200 (women) or 1500 (men).

Partner's Techniques
1. Discuss the Diet Diary with the dieter.
2. Eat all foods in designated places when around the dieter.

3. Eat only at scheduled eating times when with the dieter.

Weekly Weigh-In

Dieter's Weight _____   Date _____

Partner's Weight _____

Week Six

Throughout the sixteen-week Partnership Schedule, there will be time for review. You and your partner have used many new behaviors. You have been recording, counting calories, leaving food on the plate, eating in the same places, and heaven knows what else! It may seem at times that there is too much to learn. This week is one where my patients can use a breather— and can use time to review the techniques they have practiced in weeks past.

For week six, read over Chapters 5, 6, and 7 to learn everything there is to know about the Diet Diary and about protecting your food environment. Use this week to give each of the behaviors a full test. Discuss with your partner the problems he or she may be having. Don't forget the supportive strategies!

Techniques for the Daily Log

Dieter's Techniques

1. Fill in the Diet Diary immediately before or after eating.
2. Leave some food on your plate at each meal.
3. Do nothing else while eating.
4. Eat all food in the same place.
5. Eat all meals and snacks at scheduled times.
6. Limit calories to 1200 (women) or 1500 (men).

Partner's Techniques

1. Discuss the Diet Diary with the dieter.
2. Leave some food on your plate when with the dieter.

3. Do nothing else when eating with the dieter.
4. Eat all foods in designated places when with the dieter.
5. Eat at scheduled eating times when with the dieter.

Weekly Weigh-In

Dieter's Weight _____   Date _____
Partner's Weight _____

Week Seven

As we observed, there are three critical areas in handling food—shopping, storing, and serving meals. Preparing meals is also important, but more about that later. Keeping the landscape free of temptation can be a tremendous help to the dieter. The more you see food, the more you will want food and the more access you will have to food. You can nip this problem in the bud by keeping food out of sight. Read Chapter 8 for a description of the most prized techniques for gaining control of food cues.

Partner, you can play a major role in minimizing the dieter's contact with food. Since these cues can cause eating, decreasing the number of exposures to food can make a big difference. You can help by limiting the number of problem foods you eat in the presence of the dieter, by taking over any chores that involve dispensing food, and by assisting with food storage.

Techniques for the Daily Log

Dieter's Techniques

1. Fill out the Diet Diary immediately before or after eating.
2. Store all food out of sight.
3. Avoid being a food dispenser.
4. Remove serving dishes immediately after eating.
5. Use smaller utensils.
6. Leave the table immediately after eating.
7. Limit calories to 1200 (women) or 1500 (men).

Partner's Techniques
1. Discuss the Diet Diary with the dieter.
2. Help keep food out of sight.
3. Avoid offering food to the dieter.
4. Make sure serving dishes are removed from the table.
5. Use smaller utensils when eating with the dieter.
6. Leave the table after eating.

Weekly Weigh-In

Dieter's Weight   _____   Date _____

Partner's Weight _____

Week Eight

To eat food, one must obtain food. If the food that enters the home can be controlled, big changes can occur in eating patterns. Shopping for food can become a social event, with your partner helping before, during, or after the trip to the store. Read Chapter 8 for guidelines to harmonious shopping.

Partner, your help with the shopping can take many forms. You can help prepare the list and then check with the dieter about the foods that were purchased. You can make a tremendous contribution by doing the food shopping with the dieter or by doing the shopping for the dieter. If you aren't live-in partners, you may want to shop simultaneously but switch baskets so you each fill the other's order. Be supportive and remember to reward the dieter for making progress.

Techniques for the Daily Log

Dieter's Techniques
1. Fill out the Diet Diary immediately before or after eating.
2. Shop for food *after* eating.
3. Shop only from a list.
4. Avoid ready-to-eat foods.

5. Carry only enough money to buy items on the list.
6. Limit calories to 1200 (women) or 1500 (men).

Partner's Techniques
1. Discuss the Diet Diary with the dieter.
2. Help make a shopping list.
3. Help the dieter with the food shopping.
4. Keep ready-to-eat foods out of the house.

Weekly Weigh-In
Dieter's Weight _____   Date _____
Partner's Weight _____

Week Nine

Week nine is a review week. Since the last review week, you have learned many new behaviors. This is a lot to learn and to practice in a few short weeks, so I am using week nine to allow you to take a leisurely look at the behaviors in Chapters 7 and 8. You can decide which behaviors are right for you. Review each of the behaviors with your partner. Decide which ones merit further attention and should be saved for your stockpile of techniques.

Techniques for the Daily Log
1. Fill out the Diet Diary immediately before or after eating.
2. Store all food out of sight.
3. Avoid being a food dispenser.
4. Remove serving dishes immediately after serving.
5. Use smaller utensils.
6. Leave the table immediately after eating.
7. Shop after eating.
8. Shop only from a list.
9. Limit calories to 1200 (women) or 1500 (men).

Partner's Techniques
1. Discuss the Diet Diary with the dieter.
2. Help keep food out of sight.

3. Avoid offering food to the dieter.
4. Make sure serving dishes are removed from the table.
5. Use smaller utensils when with the dieter.
6. Help the dieter with the shopping.
7. Keep ready-to-eat foods out of the house.

Weekly Weigh-In

    Dieter's Weight ————————   Date ————

    Partner's Weight ————————

Week Ten

Eating slowly is one of the best ways to control your eating. When you eat rapidly, you consume large quantities of food before your body finds out you have had enough. This leads to overconsumption, and it also decreases your enjoyment of food (your taste buds don't have a chance when food moves by them at the speed of light!). If you slow your rate of eating, you will have time to reflect on how much you have eaten. Your body will feel full with less, and you will discover (perhaps for the first time) just how delicious some foods are.

Partner, you can help the dieter eat more slowly by slowing the pace of your eating. You may eat slowly already, in which case you don't need to slow down. If you eat rapidly, use the techniques in Chapter 9 to put the brakes on your eating pace. By modeling these behaviors, you will be setting a good example for the dieter. (Try chopsticks instead of regular utensils to convey food to your and the dieter's mouth—it takes longer!)

Techniques for the Daily Log

Dieter's Techniques

1. Fill out the Diet Diary immediately before or after eating.
2. Put your fork down between each bite.
3. Pause in the middle of the meal.

4. Limit liquids at meals.
5. Limit calories to 1200 (women) or 1500 (men).

Partner's Techniques
1. Discuss the Diet Diary with the dieter.
2. Put your fork down between bites when eating with the dieter.
3. Pause in the middle of the meal when with the dieter.
4. Help limit liquids at meals.

Weekly Weigh-In
Dieter's Weight _____   Date _____
Partner's Weight _____

Week Eleven

Your attitudes, thoughts, feelings, and emotions are important factors in your diet. These factors are ignored in almost every diet, but with the Partnership approach, you and your partner can systematically analyze and change the thoughts that influence your eating.

Motivation is the key factor in weight loss. You know what to do—doing it is the problem. When you feel frustrated, discouraged, or defeated, it is hard to stay with any program. You *can* take control of your diet thoughts. Be certain to reread Chapter 10. Focusing on thoughts is new for most dieters and requires a concerted effort.

Thoughts about dieting are not confined to the dieter. Partner, your feelings will determine how enthusiastic you are about helping the dieter. It is easy to fall prey to self-defeating thoughts and emotions. In Chapter 10 there are many procedures designed specifically for you. Practice these techniques this week.

Techniques for the Daily Log

Dieter's Techniques
1. Fill out the Diet Diary immediately before or after eating.

2. Avoid setting unreachable goals.
3. Think positively about your progress, not your shortcomings.
4. Avoid using imperatives ("always" and "never").
5. Counter dead-end thoughts with rational restatements.
6. Limit calories to 1200 (women) or 1500 (men).

Partner's Techniques
1. Discuss the Diet Diary with the dieter.
2. Help the dieter set attainable goals.
3. Discuss the dieter's thoughts about the program.
4. Counter your destructive thoughts with rational statements.

Weekly Weigh-In

Dieter's Weight _____   Date _____

Partner's Weight _____

Week Twelve

The past two weeks have included important and difficult changes. Eating slowly is foreign to most dieters and many do not part easily with their breakneck pace. More time may be needed to practice this new series of behaviors. In addition, the section on attitudes is so new, it will take several weeks to recognize the thoughts, and even longer to change them. Therefore, week twelve will be a review of the past two weeks. Read Chapters 5 and 6, and use the Daily Log to teach you which behaviors are most important.

Have you reached a weight-loss plateau? If so, don't despair. Use the methods in Chapter 6 to cope with events emotionally. Then, read Chapter 14 for crisis intervention techniques designed especially for this problem.

Spend some time this week with your partner to discuss ways that you can reward each other for moving down the path to weight loss. One enjoyable aspect of Partnership Dieting is the cooperative spirit that your mutual commitment will produce. Do some new activities together. You can use the ideas from the supportive strategies I described in Chapters 5 through 11, or you can devise your own. Show each other how much you appreciate the effort.

Techniques for the Daily Log

Dieter's Techniques

1. Fill out the Diet Diary immediately before or after eating.
2. Put your fork down between bites.
3. Pause in the middle of the meal.
4. Limit liquids at meals.
5. Avoid setting unreachable goals.
6. Think positively about progress, not shortcomings.
7. Avoid using imperatives ("always" and "never").
8. Counter dead-end thoughts with rational restatements.
9. Limit calories to 1200 (women) or 1500 (men).

Partner's Techniques

1. Discuss the Diet Diary with the dieter.
2. Put your fork down between bites when eating with the dieter.
3. Pause during the meals when with the dieter.
4. Help limit liquids at meals.
5. Help the dieter set attainable goals.
6. Discuss the dieter's thoughts about the program.
7. Counter your destructive thoughts with rational statements.

Weekly Weigh-In

Dieter's Weight _____   Date _____
Partner's Weight _____

Week Thirteen

Physical activity is crucial for your weight loss. Exercise is ignored often because it conjures up images of back-breaking calisthenics or painful laps around the track. With Partnership Dieting, increasing your physical activity is easy and painless. There are dozens of simple ways to increase physical activity. Read Chapter 11 for a description of these methods, and consult the table of caloric values for exercise in Chapter 11, to see just how many calories you can use with activities that fit into your daily routine.

Practice these simple techniques with great determination. Before long they will become permanent habits and will require no thought at all. The benefits of physical activity are far-ranging. You can enjoy improvements in your health, your emotional state, your appearance, your sleeping habits, etc. All this, just for making simple changes!

Techniques for the Daily Log

Dieter's Techniques
1. Fill out the Diet Diary immediately before or after eating.
2. Increase scheduled exercise.
3. Increase your walking.
4. Increase use of the stairs.
5. Increase other routine exercises (see Chapter 11).
6. Limit calories to 1200 (women) or 1500 (men).

Partner's Techniques
1. Discuss the Diet Diary with the dieter.
2. Help the dieter increase scheduled exercise (togetherness!).
3. Increase use of the stairs when with the dieter.
4. Increase walking when with the dieter.
5. Increase other routine activities when with the dieter.

Weekly Weigh-In
Dieter's Weight _____   Date _____
Partner's Weight _____

Week Fourteen

Since the Partnership approach to physical activity is so new for most dieters, it will take some time to acclimate yourself to these news techniques. Week fourteen will review the past week's behaviors. Plan a brainstorming session with your partner, and discuss ways to increase your routine activity. Are there ways to get more exercise at work, around the house, on your way to visit a friend, when you do the shopping, etc.?

Partnership Dieting also means Partnership Exercising! There are many ways for you and your partner to increase your physical activity and to enjoy life more. When you are at a shopping mall, use the stairs. When you take the bus downtown, you and your partner can get off several stops early and walk the extra distance. Use the opportunity to exercise to your greatest advantage by taking a walking tour of some beautiful place. There are many ways to increase your activity while you are together. Make a list of these and add them to your Daily Log.

Techniques for the Daily Log

Dieter's Techniques
1. Fill out the Diet Diary immediately before or after eating.
2. Increase your scheduled exercise.
3. Increase use of the stairs.
4. Increase your walking.
5. Increase other routine exercises.
6. Limit calories to 1200 (women) or 1500 (men).

Partner's Techniques
1. Discuss the Diet Diary with the dieter.
2. Help the dieter increase scheduled exercise.
3. Increase use of the stairs when you are with the dieter.
4. Increase walking when with the dieter.

5. Increase other routine exercises when with the dieter.

Weekly Weigh-In
>   Dieter's Weight   _____   Date _____
>   Partner's Weight _____

Week Fifteen

Week fifteen is another week to concentrate on your physical activity. You started making changes in your activity several weeks ago, so the same activities that were difficult at first are probably becoming easier. Many dieters find themselves doing more and more without even thinking about it.

As you are practicing ways to increase your exercise, you may want to view your activity with a new perspective. One of my recent patients, Roger, said it this way: "I know if I exercise I can afford to be more liberal with my eating. I buy more calories at my meals when I have exercised earlier. This helps me during the time I devote to exercise." This is a useful way of looking at physical activity for many dieters, especially those who go in for strenuous activities. However, use the calorie guide in Chapter 11 to make sure you don't consume more calories than you have earned from the exercise.

Techniques for the Daily Log

Dieter's Techniques
1. Fill out the Diet Diary immediately before or after eating.
2. Increase your scheduled exercise.
3. Increase use of the stairs.
4. Increase your walking.
5. Increase other routine activities.
6. Limit calories to 1200 (women) or 1500 (men).

Partner's Techniques
1. Discuss the Diet Diary with the dieter.
2. Help the dieter increase scheduled exercise.
3. Increase the use of stairs when with the dieter.
4. Increase walking when with the dieter.
5. Increase other routine exercises.

Weekly Weigh-In
Dieter's Weight _____   Date _____
Partner's Weight _____

Week Sixteen

You have learned an extraordinary number of techniques. Some of the changes you have made have been easy; some have been difficult. Your goal for this week is to consolidate a list of techniques that will work for *you*. You and your partner will be preparing a Permanent Daily Log that will include your most strategic techniques. In choosing these techniques, there are two other things to consider.

First, the Partnership Program is a system of principles as well as a series of techniques. The principles you have learned are of *extreme* importance. For example, you learned to remove serving dishes from the table, to store food in out-of-the-way places, and to avoid ready-to-eat foods. These techniques apply a principle—Keep Food Out of Sight. Any single technique may not be useful for you, but the principle *is*. If you learn the principle, you can apply it to your lifestyle by selecting the techniques that are relevant for you. Go back through Chapters 5 through 11 and concentrate on the principles I have described. Think of ways to apply the principles to *your* dieting situation. The behaviors that have been listed in the Daily Logs are useful for most dieters. However, the procedures *you* devise will be important, because you can best decide which procedures are most relevant.

Second, only some of the techniques you have practiced will be helpful. Some do not pertain to your lifestyle, and others are impossible for you to accomplish. This is expected, and you should remember that no dieter uses *all* the behaviors. You and your partner should have a discussion about your eating and activity patterns to determine which areas require attention. These are the areas that we will consider this week.

Partner, the same guidelines apply to you. By now you have learned many ways to help the dieter lose weight—and many ways for you to change your behavior. Reread the earlier chapters and pick out the principles of partnering I have presented. Use these principles to identify the techniques that will be most important for you and the dieter. You will be using these techniques in your Permanent Daily Log. Remember that the behaviors you have developed can be at least as useful as the techniques listed in the chapters. You are in the driver's seat, and you can best decide which procedures are critical.

The past fifteen weeks have allowed you to test new techniques, activities, and attitudes. The review weeks have been included to insure that any new procedure would receive your attention for at least two weeks. Your practice with these behaviors will provide you with the information you need to make an informed decision about the behaviors you will need for long-term success.

How do you know which behaviors are most important? The answer to this question will come from your Daily Logs, particularly the logs from the review weeks. By scanning your completed Daily Logs, you will form a picture of the techniques that were associated with weight change. From your point totals you will see which behaviors were easiest to mold into your daily schedule. Look back over the "Techniques for the Daily Log" for each week (in this chapter). Select the techniques that are most important for you. Add any new techniques you developed yourself. Your final list should contain no fewer than five behaviors and no more than twelve behaviors (any more is a burden).

Use your composite list of techniques to form the Permanent Daily Log. The Permanent Log will be made from the blank Daily Log presented earlier in this chapter. Make copies of the blank Daily Log and enter the behaviors from your list of important techniques. The Permanent Daily Log will contain only those behaviors that are helpful for you. The Permanent Daily Log will always include an item on filling out the Diet Diary and an item for totaling your calories for each day. These two items will form the backbone of your program.

Techniques for the Daily Log

Dieter's Techniques
1. Fill out the Diet Diary immediately before or after eating.
2. Limit calories to 1200 (women) or 1500 (men).

    (Add the techniques you have chosen from the past Daily Logs. Select the techniques that are most important.)

Partner's Techniques

1. Discuss the Diet Diary with the dieter.
   (Add the techniques you have chosen from the past Daily Logs. Select the techniques that are most important.)

Weekly Weigh-In
    Dieter's Weight _____   Date _____
    Partner's Weight _____

PART **3**

Crisis Control
Techniques

There are two crisis situations that every dieter confronts: special events where eating is the main'event *(weddings, Thanksgiving, etc.), and a weight plateau (no matter what you do, you can't lose weight). The time has passed when these crisis situations can throw your diet into a tailspin. The Partnership Program has special crisis intervention techniques to put* you *in control.*

CHAPTER 13

Coping with Special Occasions: Anti-Orgy Techniques

CRISIS ALERT: Holiday, party, or feast ahead!

CRISIS INTERVENTION: Anti-orgy techniques (making sure the turkey is the only one stuffed on Thanksgiving).

Dieters have a love-hate relationship with invitations to parties, weddings, holiday feasts, reunions, company picnics, and so forth. They are pleased with the prospect of a gala social event, but are plunged into gloom by the fear of the inevitable eating orgy. An eating orgy exacts a painful toll—not only do calories skyrocket for the day, but the guilt of overindulgence can linger for weeks.

This chapter will arm you with an array of techniques designed to meet the challenge of special events. You deserve to enjoy festive occasions—without the fear that food will get the best of you. These techniques will allow you to eat (without going on a binge), drink (in moderation), and be merry (you can celebrate your weight loss).

Partner, these crisis situations are ready-made for your support. You will have many food-control procedures at your disposal to help the dieter through difficult times. There are specific techniques you both can use to insure that special events do not become traumatic events.

169

To cope with special events, you must prepare yourself psychologically and behaviorally. You and your partner will learn behavioral procedures to master even the most difficult events. Psychological preparation is just as important. If you are unprepared psychologically, you can have real problems before, during, and after a special event. The importance of emotional factors is illustrated in these two case studies. As you read the cases, see if you can identify the areas where coping skills would have helped.

Harriet and Bill were invited to a June wedding. Harriet was in a frenzy by early May. Her 175 pounds would never look good in a party dress, and her relatives hadn't seen her since she weighed 145. She was determined to lose fifteen pounds before she bought a dress, and to lose the remaining fifteen pounds before the wedding. Harriet's "starvation" diet included one slice of toast and black coffee for breakfast, cottage cheese for lunch, and two hard-boiled eggs for supper. She was irritable and felt deprived because she was hungry all day and because she still prepared conventional meals for Bill.

Harriet lost five pounds during the first week. Instead of feeling good, Harriet dwelled on the twenty-five pounds she still had to lose. She dreamed about food at night, thought about food during the day, and made Bill miserable with her irritability and complaints. By the time of the wedding she had lost only seven pounds.

At the wedding Harriet was so sure everyone was talking about her weight that she decided to drown her misery in food. She felt so guilty afterward that she cried herself to sleep that night. Worst of all, Harriet did not wake up the next morning determined to start a sensible weight-loss program. She used her misguided experience as further proof that she couldn't manage to stay on a diet. It wasn't long before Harriet had eaten her way back to 175—and more.

Ellen also wanted to diet; the day after Thanksgiving would be her first day. Her reasoning: "I know I'll eat too much on Thanksgiving, so even if I started now I'd surely blow it then. I might as well put it off until after the holiday."

You can predict what happened. Not only did the holiday become an occasion for overeating, but the whole month before was a nonstop feast. "I might as well enjoy myself now," Ellen kept telling herself, "because I suffer when I start to diet." Ellen was in the classic double bind. She had decided to diet the day after Thanksgiving, but her month of overeating added ten pounds to the amount she needed to lose. She was beaten even before she had started.

These two examples underscore the importance of your attitude in preparing for special events. Vowing to lose weight for a specific event (like a wedding) can lead to trouble. There may be too much weight to lose in too little time, and the struggle against an impossible goal only breeds frustration. When Harriet received the wedding invitation, she should have said, "I know I can't lose all the weight before the wedding, and I know how miserable I am when I starve myself. I will start the program now and then continue to diet sensibly after the wedding." Ellen could have coped with the impending holiday by saying, "If I start dieting now, I won't feel guilty about enjoying myself on Thanksgiving. After all, one bad day doesn't ruin a good diet."

The first step in coping with a special event is to maintain constant surveillance over your thoughts and attitudes. The techniques described in Chapter 10 will help you deal with special events before and after they occur. Now we can concentrate on coping strategies to be used *during* the event. Here is your orgy insurance.

Anti-Orgy Techniques

Social events can be the downfall of many dieters. No more! These techniques will show you and your partner how to mastermind a carefully detailed plan to transform a difficult situation into a joyous occasion.

Sit with Your Partner

Your partner can ease the strain of a social event with support and words of praise. If the occasion demands that you and your partner be separated, arrange a set of long-distance signals.

Shirley described this scene at a big family wedding: "Jim was terrific. He knows my weakness is bread and butter, so he asked for the bread basket each time he saw it on my side of the table. People wondered why he never took any bread, but he kept the basket at his side until someone asked for it." Jim also caught Shirley's eye frequently throughout the meal, smiling and nodding his pleasure at how well she was doing. This support was important to her.

Partner: Before you go to a social event, have a strategy session to decide where the booby traps are likely to be. Then you can plan ways to help the dieter avoid problem foods. You might be in charge of getting the drinks, so the dieter will have low-calorie beverages. If you will be ordering food, plan with the dieter what each of you will eat, and then *you* place the orders. Remember that events with unlimited food can be agonizing for the dieter. Your praise and support can be just the boost the dieter needs.

Have Your Partner Fill Your Plate at a Buffet

Some of my patients are demoralized by platter after platter of hot and cold calories. The buffet gauntlet can be the undoing of even the most well-planned meals. Your partner can wait on you by ferrying your plate between you and the buffet. When your partner returns with the food, discuss the calorie values to see if your partner has made prudent (but delicious) choices.

Partner: A hint for dressing up the dieter's plate: serve the dieter small portions of many foods. The different tastes will give the dieter just as much pleasure as large quantities of a few foods. Select some foods the dieter may not have tried before. The novelty can overpower the need for quantity. If you are planning to make several trips to the buffet, start with low-calorie foods (soup, carrot or celery sticks, etc.) to begin the meal. When the high-calorie foods are served, the dieter will not be famished.

Plan Your Meal in Advance

Sit down with your partner to plan an eating strategy for the special event. List every item on the menu and write down the calories for typical servings of each food. Remember, there is nothing you can't eat—as long as you count the calories in your daily total.

Determining what foods will be served may not be easy. There is no problem if the hostess is a relative or a close friend. You may suffer from a twinge of embarrassment if the hostess is not a close acquaintance, but the effort will pay off when you appear at the event with a plan of attack. Betsy is allergic to crabmeat, so she never hesitated to ask about the contents of the menu. She even queries banquet managers when she is invited to an event in a hotel or a catering hall.

Here is an example of how you can plan for a typical banquet at a wedding, anniversary party, or other catered event. You first inquire to find that the meal will include fruit cup, consommé, roast beef, baked potato, string beans and mushrooms, ice cream with chocolate sauce, coffee, and cookies. Except for the dessert, it seems harmless, doesn't it? But when you do the calorie count you find out differently.

One meal and you are already 400 calories over your day's allotment—without allowing for breakfast and lunch. On a past diet you might have eliminated the potato, bread, butter, dessert, cream and sugar, and the cookies. You would have been left with 856 calories—and a very de-

Food	Amount	Calories
Fruit cup	½ cup	126
Consommé	1 cup	22
Roast beef (lean rib roast)	10 oz.	688
Baked potato	4¾ in.	145
Butter for potato	2 pats	70
String beans & mushrooms	½ cup	20
Italian bread	2 slices	56
Butter for bread	2 pats	70
Vanilla ice cream	½ cup	138
shredded coconut	2 tbsp.	66
chocolate syrup	2 tbsp.	92
Coffee with cream and sugar	1 cup	47
Cookies	2	100
	TOTAL	1640

prived feeling. If you had just eliminated dessert, you would have consumed 1244 calories, even if you didn't have a single drink!

On the Partnership Diet Program, you and your partner decide what you will eat and exactly how many calories you will have. You won't be deprived and you won't feel guilty about overeating. Here is one preplanned way to cope with this banquet.

Together with your partner, you ponder cutting out the fruit cup. You decide that starting the meal by fiddling with your napkin while everybody else eats will put you at a disadvantage. You then plan to eat half of the fruit cup (63 calories) and all of the consommé (a bargain at 22 calories). You have had two courses for less than 100 calories, and you have taken the edge off your appetite.

Now for the main course. You decide that four ounces of roast beef (275 calories) is plenty. This will let you have the roast beef you really love without sabotaging your calorie total. If you eat half of the potato (73) with one pat of butter (35) and the vegetable (20), you will have had a total of only 488 calories. If you forgo the bread and butter, you can eat the ice cream sundae (296) and have black coffee (0), for a grand total of 784 calories. And I do mean grand! Try telling the person sitting next to you that you are on a diet, then put away a complete meal of fruit, soup, roast beef, buttered potato, vegetable, and ice cream sundae with chocolate syrup, and watch for the response! This is suffering?!

At just under 800 calories, you have enough left over to manage a poached egg (81) on cinnamon-raisin bread (62) for breakfast. For lunch you could have tuna salad from 2 ounces of tuna (75) with a teaspoon of mayonnaise (34) stuffed into a fresh tomato (20), along with a six-ounce glass of skim milk (66).

The total for the day—1123 calories. Add 85 calories for a 3½ ounce glass of wine, or champagne to toast the bride, and you have still managed to sail through a difficult day at 1208 calories!

Would you have planned this differently? You could trade half of the dessert for two Scotch-and-waters (220), or for two slices of Italian bread (56) and two pats of butter (70). You're the boss. This system can work because *you* are in control. See how easy it is?

Eat Something before the Event

Don't arrive on an empty stomach. If you are attending a wedding breakfast, a midday holiday feast, or a nighttime gala, eat something first. Dieters are often tempted to skip lunch before a midafternoon or evening event. It is best to have a few celery stalks, some carrot sticks, a tossed salad, or perhaps a cup of bouillon with a slice of toast. You will be calmer about the array of food at the special event, and you will probably consume fewer calories in the long run.

Eat More Slowly than Anyone at the Table

Slowing your eating will make you feel full with less food. Use the techniques from Chapter 9. Put your fork down between bites and pause during the meal. Try to be the last one to pick up the fork when the meal begins. By pacing yourself, you can be the last one to finish. Your partner can help by setting a slow pace and by showing some support when you are able to slow your eating. This will shorten those stretches between courses when you might otherwise be tempted to raid the bread basket.

Strategic Defenses for Other Events

Some events are particularly troublesome. Cocktail parties, for example, are loaded with powerful aliments. Emergency measures are necessary to emerge from these events with your virtue intact.

Cocktail Parties

Most cocktail parties have everything to drink and nothing to eat (except peanuts, pretzels, potato chips, and other high-calorie specialties). The best defense is to eat beforehand and to prepare for the liquid calories you will consume. Plan your preparty meal with your partner, and plan the number and type of drinks you will have.

The calorie guide in Appendix A will show you which drinks have the fewest calories. A white wine spritzer made with two ounces of wine (48 calories) and club soda (0) will last as long as a Scotch-and-water and will give you only half the calories. Beware of high-calorie drinks like sweet vermouth and cream sherry (180–200 calories for four ounces), and of regular mixers like tonic water, ginger ale, and fruit drinks (76–113 calories for eight ounces). Quench your thirst with water, diet soda, club soda, Bloody Mary mix, and so forth, *before* you start with the alcoholic beverages. Many dieters bring their own diet soda to cocktail parties.

Office Parties

Unless you work at a stylish place, a celebration at the office may involve pretzels and potato chips eaten from a box, along with wine, beer, or hard liquor served in paper cups. How do you cope?

If your partner is a co-worker, plan to take over the "refreshments committee." Along with the high-calorie foods, you can buy foods that will not send your diet into a tailspin. Or bring your own. You can include bottles of diet soda and fresh fruit. You could even bring some Magic Dip (see Chapter 16) and a bag of carrot sticks and radishes. Avoid being on the "clean-up committee." This way you won't be encouraged to eat the remaining food or to take it home with you.

Your Own Parties

Regina had trouble with her weight because she loved to entertain and she couldn't resist eating her own good cooking. Finally, she agreed to try an experiment: the next time she had guests, she served the sensible and delicious dishes she was learning to cook for herself and her fiancé. She was surprised by the positive response to marinated mushrooms instead of quiche, herb-broiled chicken instead of a dish with a rich sauce, and a fresh fruit salad instead of chocolate mousse. Even people who are not dieting like to be served a light and tasty meal instead of a procession of heavy dishes. They will never guess they are eating "diet food."

Partner, you can help with parties by sitting down with the dieter to plan the meals. You may want to use the dishes in Chapter 16, or you can use the calorie guides in the appendixes to prepare your own creative dishes. The dieter's burden can also be eased if you help with the shopping, preparation, and serving of the meals.

CHAPTER 14

How to Get Off a Weight Plateau: The Three-Day Morale-Booster Crisis Diet

CRISIS ALERT: The needle on your scale is stuck! You stayed within your calorie allowance. You may have even increased your physical activity, but the scale shows no loss, or even worse, a weight gain.

CRISIS INTERVENTION: *The Three-Day Morale-Booster Crisis Diet.*

Laura was discouraged because she had dieted religiously for seven straight days. She played tennis one day and rode her bicycle another. To her surprise, she had gained two pounds. Her reaction? "What's the use of dieting if I don't lose weight? I feel like giving up." My reaction? "Chin up, Laura! I have a three-day plan that will show your scale who's boss."

I know how discouraging it can be to get stuck on a weight plateau. The plateau can also be discouraging for your partner. You can put your mind at ease, because there is a crisis intervention plan designed specifically for this problem. This plan will get your weight loss moving again and will improve your spirits so you can adhere to the program with Herculean determination. You will be interrupting your 1200- to 1500-calorie plan for just three days (no more). When the weight begins dropping, you can return to your customary eating patterns.

Partner, if *you* think a weight plateau is discouraging, just think how the dieter feels. This is the time when you and the dieter need a powerful technique, like the Morale-Booster Diet. The diet is so novel that you may want to use it yourself, especially if you are watching your weight. Study the diet with the dieter, and share in as many of the meals as possible. This will help the dieter make the appropriate food choices for the three-day plan and will help boost the dieter's morale by your visible show of support.

Before starting the diet, it is important to identify the causes of your weight plateau. Your weight may have been halted by omissions in the program or by natural causes. Have you been conscientious about counting calories and about weighing portions? Have you been overlooking those easy-to-forget calories like the dressing on your salad, the ketchup on your hamburger, or the mayonnaise on your sandwich? Each instance of eating amnesia can have a small effect until one day you will be surprised by the scale.

If you can rule out these errors of omission, look to natural causes to explain the plateau. Here are two factors that can create day-to-day fluctuations in your weight.

1. *Salt intake and your water balance.* Slight changes in your water balance can have a great influence on your body weight, and salt plays an important role in regulating your water balance. In women, 55 percent of total body weight is water, and in men, 59 percent is water. A small accumulation of water (edema) or a small water loss (dehydration) can lead to dramatic weight changes. Fad diets that promote instant weight loss sometimes promote dehydration by curtailing salt intake. The weight loss is temporary, and the process can be dangerous.

If you have reached a weight plateau, you may have made changes in your salt intake without knowing it. You may be losing fat, but the increased water retention may mask your loss. This does *not* mean that you should change the amount of salt in your diet. It does mean that fluctuations in your weight are to be expected. If you suspect problems with water retention, consult your physician.

2. *Hormonal influences on body weight.* Many of my female patients report gaining as much as five pounds around the time of menstruation. Hormonal changes during the menstrual cycle can influence water retention, causing body weight to increase at a discouraging rate. The same phenomenon can occur if you are taking birth control pills or estrogen replacement medication for menopause.

There is no need to change your diet if you are eating sensibly and nutritiously. Your body will eventually regulate its water level. You can help by being patient and by not succumbing to despair.

If you are marooned on a weight plateau, you need innovative measures. These techniques can turn the tide, and you will eat well in the process.

The Three-Day Morale-Booster Crisis Diet

The Morale-Booster Diet is easy to follow. It is low in calories (approximately 800 each day) and has sufficient protein and nutrients to be fairly well balanced. You will start to lose weight again, and then you can return to your basic meal plans. The diet contains adequate nutrition, but I advise you to supplement it with a multiple vitamin pill each day to insure that you have *all* the vitamins you need.

The diet is *not* to be followed for more than three days. Remember that you need to be eating the foods that you enjoy and can live with for a lifetime. This diet is only for the plateau crisis. After the three days elapse, you *must* go back to your 1200- or 1500-calorie regimen to continue losing weight gradually and steadily. (If you have special dietary requirements be sure to check with your physician to make sure this diet meets your needs.)

The Morale-Booster Diet is designed to provide structure in a time of crisis. You may vary the foods any way you like, as long as you do not eat or drink anything that is not on the diet.

This plan allows you a total of sixty ounces of liquids and/or solids each day. Every day of the diet is different, so you will have a variety of delicious foods. Day one contains liquids only, except for diet gelatin. On day two you will exchange eight ounces of liquids for eight ounces of meat or fish. On day three you exchange another eight ounces of liquids for eight ounces of raw vegetables.

Partner, you can make certain the Morale-Booster Diet goes well for the dieter by doing several things before the diet even starts. Sit down with the dieter and plan to buy the necessary foods and beverages for the three-day period. If you can do the shopping with the dieter, the diet will get off to an enthusiastic start. If the dieter prepares meals for the family, you can help with preparation or serving of the foods, so the dieter will minimize contact with foods that are not on the list. It may also help to rid the house of problem foods that are not part of the diet.

Now that both of you are prepared for a boost in morale, Ready, Set, GO!

Day One

Select a total of sixty ounces from the following choices (no substitutions allowed) in any combination you prefer:

Skim milk	11 calories per ounce
Unsweetened grapefruit juice	12 calories per ounce
Tomato juice	6 calories per ounce
Diet gelatin	2 calories per ounce

Just wait until you see the delicious ways you can use these foods!

Day Two

Select fifty-two ounces from the same choices, again in any combination. Add eight ounces of lean meat (beef, chicken, or liver) or fish, baked or broiled, to total sixty ounces for the day.

> Lean meat (beef, chicken, liver) 40–60 calories per ounce
> Fish (broiled or baked)   20–55 calories per ounce

Day Three

Select forty-four ounces from the day one choices, in any combination. Add eight ounces of meat or fish, as in day two. In addition, add eight ounces of mixed raw vegetables, making your selection from this list:

Bean sprouts	Green peppers
Beets	Lettuce
Broccoli	Mushrooms
Carrots	Radishes
Cauliflower	Spinach
Celery	Tomatoes
Cucumbers	Zucchini

Vegetables can be dressed with lemon juice or vinegar. Once again, your day's total is sixty ounces. As with day one and day two, some of the ounces are fluid ounces and some are weight ounces. Don't let this confuse you; for the purposes of this diet, they are interchangeable.

Every Day

Drink as much water, diet soda, unsweetened or artificially sweetened coffee or tea as you like. The milk you put in your coffee is part of your day's allowance. Meat and fish may be seasoned with lemon juice or mustard as desired, and milk may be flavored with extracts. Use no butter or margarine.

Orchestrating This Diet

Does skim milk bore you? Turn to the recipes for Dreamy Whipped Topping, Hot Choco-Mocha and Spoon-

Licking Milk Shakes in Chapter 16, to see a few of the creative ways you can use milk. Eight ounces of skim milk makes enough topping to cover portion after portion of diet gelatin with indescribable sweetness. You won't believe you are on a diet.

Hot Choco-Mocha isn't fattening—just delicious. The mocha and an entire repertoire of thick milkshakes can be whipped up with the aid of flavored extracts. At an average 10 calories per teaspoon, these extracts (chocolate, rum, almond, vanilla, etc.) will not have an appreciable effect on your total calorie count.

Diet gelatin is your only "solid" food on day one, but it can be a special treat when you make it disappear under a mountain of Whipped Topping. Count each half-cup serving of gelatin as four ounces.

The following sample menus show you how deliciously you can eat on the Morale-Booster Diet . . . even on day one, with just four basic ingredients.

Hard to believe, isn't it? Try explaining to your friends that you are actually losing weight by eating and drinking all these wonderful foods.

Again, follow this regimen for only three days. After you complete the Morale-Booster Diet, go back to your 1200- or 1500-calorie meal plans. Now that you have passed the hurdle of an interrupted weight loss, you can progress to your weight-loss goal.

DAY ONE MENU

		Ounces	Calories
BREAKFAST	Grapefruit juice, 2 5-oz. glasses	10	120
	Coffee with skim milk (1 oz.)	1	11
MIDMORNING SNACK*	Banana milk shake** (6 oz. milk)	6	66
LUNCH	Tomato juice, 4-oz. glass	4	24
	Cherry diet gelatin (1 cup = 8 oz.)	8	16
	with Whipped Topping (2 oz. milk)	2	22
MIDAFTERNOON SNACK*	Hot chocolate** 1 tbsp. cocoa with		14
	6 oz. skim milk, and	6	66
	Whipped Topping** (2 oz. milk)	2	22
DINNER	Tomato juice, 4-oz. glass	4	24
	Coffee milk shake** (6 oz. milk)	6	66
BEDTIME SNACK*	Raspberry diet gelatin (1 cup = 8 oz.)	8	16
	with Whipped Topping (2 oz. milk)	2	22
	TOTAL	59	489

On day two, divide your meat and fish between two meals and really feast!

DAY TWO MENU

		Ounces	Calories
BREAKFAST	Grapefruit juice, 2 5-oz. glasses	10	120
	Coffee milk shake** (6 oz. milk)	6	66
MIDMORNING SNACK*	Raspberry diet gelatin (1 cup = 8 oz.)	8	48
	with Whipped Topping (2 oz. milk)	2	22
	Jasmine tea		0
LUNCH	Tomato juice, 2 4-oz. glasses	8	48
	Broiled fish (4 oz.), lemon juice	4	135
	Diet soda or coffee		0
MIDAFTERNOON SNACK*	Maple Walnut milk shake** (6 oz. milk)	6	66
DINNER	Broiled Chicken	4	155
	with tomato sauce** (2 oz.)	2	24
BEDTIME SNACK*	Hot chocolate** 1 tbsp. cocoa		14
	with 6 oz. milk	6	66
	with Whipped Topping (2 oz. milk)	2	22
	TOTAL	58	786

On day three, add the satisfying crunch of fresh vegetables to your menu.

DAY THREE MENU

		Ounces	Calories
BREAKFAST	Tomto juice, 2 4-oz. glasses	8	48
	Coffee with skim milk (1 oz.)	1	11
MIDMORNING SNACK*	Chocolate mint milk shake** (6 oz. milk)	6	66
	with 1 tbsp. cocoa		14
LUNCH	Broiled hamburger (lean 4 oz.)	4	250
	Mixed vegetable salad (4 oz.)	4	40
	Diet soda, coffee, tea		0
MIDAFTERNOON SNACK*	Café au lait** (4 oz. milk)	4	44
DINNER	Grapefruit juice, 1 5-oz. glass	5	60
	Broiled fish (4 oz.), mustard sauce	4	135
	Mixed vegetable salad (4 oz.)	4	40
	Coffee milk shake** (6 oz. milk)	6	66
BEDTIME SNACK*	Strawberry diet gelatin (1 cup = 8 oz.)	8	48
	with Whipped Topping (2 oz. milk)	2	22
	Rum toddy** (4 oz. milk)	4	44
	TOTAL	60	888

* Use snacks if part of your established eating schedule. If not, budget extra foods for mealtimes.
** See recipe index.

PART **4**

Increasing Your Weight-Loss Wisdom

Learn all *of the important facts about dieting by taking the Weight-Loss Wisdom Test. Then feast your eyes on delectable Magic Recipes and on 124 menus that include your favorite foods!*

CHAPTER 15

Diet Facts and Fallacies: Testing Your Weight-Loss Wisdom

Now you can show off your nutrition know-how and your exercise acumen. This quiz contains answers to the most frequently asked questions about dieting. Take this quiz with your partner to see which of you can boast of the greater weight-loss wisdom. The quiz is a real challenge. You may find that some of your most cherished diet "facts" are actually fallacies.

Is it bad to eat large quantities of food just before you go to bed? Is honey a better sweetener than sugar? How can you rid yourself of cellulite? Does grapefruit help burn fat? You are about to find the answers to these and many more important questions about dieting.

Answer each question by marking "true" or "false." Correct answers and explanations for each question will follow. At the end of the chapter you can see how your score compares to the scores of other aspiring dieters.

TEST FOR WEIGHT-LOSS WISDOM

	True	False
1. Skipping meals is a good way to lose weight.	———	———
2. It is snacks that are fattening, not regular meals.	———	———

	True	*False*
3. If you eat less at each meal, your stomach will shrink and you won't feel as hungry.	____	____
4. Excess weight is caused by excess water, so taking water pills is a good way to lose weight.	____	____
5. Even if an overweight person feels perfectly healthy, the excess weight can be dangerous.	____	____
6. If you continue to eat the same amount of food each year, you will gradually put on weight as you grow older.	____	____
7. An overweight person who loses weight and then gains it back is no worse off than before the weight was lost.	____	____
8. The tendency to be fat is inherited. If a person's parents are both fat, it is unlikely that he or she will be able to lose weight.	____	____
9. Fat people are gluttons.	____	____
10. If you adhere strictly to a diet and don't "cheat," you will lose weight every week.	____	____
11. Eating before bedtime is bad because the body cannot burn the calories as fast.	____	____
12. Natural foods are not necessarily useful for a diet.	____	____

	True	False
13. There is no need for dieters to take vitamin pills every day.	___	___
14. Starches are fattening and should be avoided.	___	___
15. A couple of drinks can't hurt; it's just liquid.	___	___
16. Potatoes are not fattening.	___	___
17. Margarine is just as fattening as butter.	___	___
18. Plain yogurt is good for a diet.	___	___
19. Grapefruit helps to burn fat.	___	___
20. Toast has fewer calories than bread.	___	___
21. Whole wheat bread and white bread are about equal in calories.	___	___
22. Washing spaghetti and rice lowers the calories	___	___
23. Honey is a better sweetener than sugar.	___	___
24. Expensive cuts of beef are more fattening than inexpensive cuts.	___	___
25. Sugarless gum has just as many calories as regular gum.	___	___
26. Dieters can eat unlimited amounts of vegetables because they are so low in calories.	___	___
27. High-fiber foods will speed your weight loss.	___	___

28. The best diet is very low in carbo-hydrates.

29. High-fat foods are good for a diet because they help curb your appetite.

30. Exercise is not helpful for dieting because it increases your appetite.

31. Health spas may not be good places to lose weight.

32. A fat baby is a healthy baby.

33. Children usually do not outgrow their "baby fat."

34. Breast-fed babies are less likely to be fat than bottle-fed babies.

35. Children should be allowed to have sweets or they will develop an abnormal craving later on.

36. Natural sugar is no better for you than refined sugar.

37. Overweight people are more likely to have psychological problems than slim people.

38. It is impossible to reduce in certain spots by exercising or by eating certain foods.

39. The liquid protein diet is safe and effective.

40. It is important to count the calories in ketchup, mayonnaise, and other condiments when on a diet.

41. The more vitamins and proteins you consume, the better off you will be.   ____   ____

42. There is no evidence that oysters, eggs, red meat, or vitamin E can increase virility.   ____   ____

43. Those ugly lumps of fat are cellulite, and need to be broken up.   ____   ____

Answers and Explanations

1. FALSE. Many dieters try to cut calories by skipping breakfast and even lunch, then are so famished by dinnertime they consume more food than if they had eaten moderately throughout the day. Some people regard the "martyrdom" of missed meals as a license to go on a binge later.

Aside from the futility of this starve-and-stuff routine, skipping meals has unfavorable metabolic consequences regardless of the number of calories consumed. Research has shown that taking one big meal a day is associated with increased fat production, elevated cholesterol, and impaired glucose tolerance. You may actually add more fat than if you have the same number of calories spread over three meals. There is evidence that fat people *do* tend to eat *fewer* meals in a day than thin people.

2. FALSE. Whether you call your food a meal or a snack, if you consume more calories than your body needs, you will gain weight. Snacking between meals may help some people eat less later and therefore can be helpful in a weight-loss program. For others, it is a hindrance. Analyze your own eating behavior to decide if snacking should be a planned part of your diet.

3. FALSE. Your stomach does not "shrink." It *is* true, however, that if you eat smaller meals for a long period of time you will feel full with less food in your stomach. This phenomenon is not clearly understood and may well be psychological.

4. FALSE. Water makes up a smaller percentage of body weight in an overweight person than in a normal-weight person. Water pills (diuretics) can dangerously dehydrate an overweight person and are not indicated for weight loss. It is also unwise to avoid drinking fluids in an attempt to lose weight. The effect is temporary at best, and may be dangerous. If you suspect you are one of the *small* number of people who have water retention problems, be sure to see your doctor.

5. TRUE. Excess weight is implicated in a number of very serious medical problems, the most important being heart disease. With some of these problems you may not notice any symptoms at all. For example, many people with high blood pressure feel fine, yet high blood pressure is a major risk factor for heart disease.

6. TRUE. As you grow older your body requires less energy to satisfy its metabolic needs—about 5 percent less every ten years, starting at age thirty-five. Also, people tend to become less active as they age. If your food intake remains constant while your energy requirements and your energy expenditure decrease, weight gain will be the inevitable result.

7. FALSE. Research indicates that losing and regaining weight repeatedly may be *more* harmful than simply *staying* overweight. Blood pressure and serum cholesterol tend to be high in overweight people, and they can increase abnormally during periods of weight *gain*. In studies with animals, repeated episodes of dramatic weight loss followed by rapid weight gain have been associated with serious heart problems.

There is another complication: when you lose weight rapidly, especially without exercising, you lose lean body tissue as well as fat, because the body is not able to mobilize its fat stores quickly enough. When you regain the weight rapidly, the body cannot produce lean tissue as quickly as fat, so much of the excess energy is converted to fat. Every time the reduce-regain pattern is repeated, this up-and-down pattern creates psychological hazards: it is disheartening to suffer through a series of aborted diets.

8. FALSE. Research on the genetics of obesity is just now being conducted on humans, so we still are not sure to what degree obesity is inherited. Man has known for thousands of years that domestic animals can be bred to be fat, and many people feel that obesity is equally inheritable in humans. For example, if a child has one overweight parent, there is a 40 percent chance he will also be overweight. If both parents are overweight, the chances increase to 80 percent. It is possible that weight problems are inherited. However, overweight parents may teach their children poor eating habits, may always have fattening foods available, and may pass along food preferences that contribute to obesity.

The best argument against the inevitability of obesity is that some offspring of fat parents do manage to take weight off and keep it off successfully.

9. FALSE. Most overweight people do eat more than normal-weight people, but not so voraciously that they deserve to be called gluttons. More notably, nearly all overweight people are less active than thin people, so the energy they do consume is less likely to be used.

10. FALSE. Nearly every dieter reaches a plateau at some point in a weight-loss regimen. A number of factors—for example, water retention—can halt weight loss temporarily. The dieter should be aware of feelings that the program is ineffective. This can lead to loss of hope and a return to the old patterns of eating. If you stay with the program, the pounds will start coming off again.

11. FALSE. The body is a simple machine. It takes in energy through eating and expends it through activity. *What* and *how much* you eat are what count, not the time of day. Like your bank account, your fat stores depend on the balance of deposits and withdrawals, not the timing.

12. TRUE. Eating natural foods—those grown organically or prepared without additives or preservatives—may be a sound nutritional practice, because some additives may be harmful. All the evidence isn't in yet. However, "natural" does not mean "low-calorie." On the contrary, some nut mixes, special cereals, and other foods found in natural-food stores are very high in calories.

13. TRUE. It is important to eat a balanced diet any time, not just while you are on a diet. There is probably no need to take a vitamin supplement if you choose a variety of foods from the essential groups—meats and other proteins, breads and cereals, milk and milk products, fruits and vegetables. Vitamins are usually recommended in conjunction with various "crash" diets because important nutrients are often missing from these unbalanced diets. Such a dangerous weight-loss regimen is not recommended, with or without vitamins.

14. FALSE. Starches (complex carbohydrates) and proteins contain 4½ calories per gram. So gram for gram, starch is no more "fattening" than protein. Fats, which contain 9 calories per gram, are the culprit. You do not necessarily need to decrease the amount of starch you eat, unless it makes up a disproportionate part of your daily diet. It is important to eat the right kinds of starch—those that are high in fiber. Pasta has little fiber, while corn, potatoes, dried beans, and peas are high in fiber. The legumes—beans, peas, lentils—provide good nutrition (including protein) at low cost.

15. FALSE. Alcohol is high in calories and mixed drinks can be even higher. (See the calorie table in Appendix A.) For example, a Tom Collins has 180 calories and a Manhattan 165. Beer is one of the better calorie bargains at 101 calories for eight ounces (the "light" beers are even lower in calories), as is white wine at 90 calories for four ounces.

16. TRUE. One medium-sized boiled potato contains only 75 calories, and a small baked potato has only about 95 calories. However, adding a quarter-cup of sour cream doubles the calories, and two tablespoons of butter or margarine more than triples the count. Frying potatoes boosts the calorie count because of the oil you consume.

17. TRUE. Margarine and butter are equivalent in calories: 100 per tablespoon. However, there is one major difference between the two: butter is primarily animal (saturated) fat while margarine is primarily vegetable (unsaturated) fat. Saturated fats tend to raise blood cholesterol and promote the deposit of fatty substances on the walls of your arteries (a major factor in heart disease). Unsaturated fats tend to lower cholesterol. Margarine is, therefore, the better choice. Safflower oil produces the greatest cholesterol-lowering effect, followed by corn oil, soybean oil, cottonseed oil, and sunflower oil.

Baylor College of Medicine's Help Your Heart Eating Plan suggests that you consume two tablespoons of unsaturated fat each day. It is easy to do this by cooking with safflower or corn oil.

18. TRUE. An eight-ounce serving of plain, unflavored yogurt has twelve grams of protein, four grams of fat, and only 150 calories. This is a high ratio of protein to fat, and the calories are reasonable. You can cut the calories even further by making your own yogurt with low-fat skim milk. However, the fruit-flavored yogurts are fairly high in calories—usually about 250 or more per cup—so a container of yogurt can use up a fifth of your daily allotment. Add your own fruit, low-calorie preserves, wheat germ, artificial sweetener, or other flavorings to plain yogurt, instead of buying the fruit-flavored varieties.

19. FALSE. Ever since the first "Grapefruit Diet" appeared back in the thirties, mystical fat-burning qualities have been attributed to grapefruit. Some people think they can eat *anything* and still lose weight, as long as they begin each meal with a grapefruit. Grapefruit is delicious, supplies vitamin C, is low in calories and carbohydrates, and provides more bulk than citrus juices. This explains why it appears in nearly every diet. However, it has no special fat-burning qualities. There is no magical food that will "burn off fat." The way to get rid of fat is to use more energy than you take in.

20. FALSE. Toast removes some water but no calories. Let your preference dictate your choice, because it has no effect on your diet.

21. TRUE. Whole wheat bread has a higher fiber content and for this reason may be a wiser choice. But the calorie difference is negligible.

22. FALSE. Washing these foods before cooking removes only a minuscule amount of starch and almost no calories. It does, however, remove some of the vitamins.

23. FALSE. Honey has 65 calories per tablespoon, sugar 45. Since honey is a more efficient sweetener, you may need to use a little less honey than sugar for the same sweetening effect. In actual use the calorie count will probably turn out to be equivalent. Many people think of honey as a "health food," but honey and sugar are nutritionally equivalent. The choice is one of preference.

24. TRUE. Expensive cuts are expensive because they taste better and are more tender. This is due to "marbling" —streaks of fat throughout the meat. Inexpensive cuts are likely to be leaner (after you cut off the fat around the edges) and therefore will have fewer calories per ounce.

25. TRUE. Carbohydrates in sugarless gums can bring the calorie total to 7 or 8 or more—just about the same as regular gum. Check your brand's label for the exact information.

26. FALSE. Vegetables differ greatly in their calorie values. Many are excellent calorie buys—although *any-thing* eaten to excess can hinder your diet. Others are not such great calorie bargains. The following vegetables should be included in your diet for their nutritional benefits, but only in limited quantities. (Calories shown are for a half-cup serving; the range takes into account type—frozen, canned, fresh—and stage of cooking—boiled, baked, mashed, etc.)

"Limited" vegetables	*Calories per ½ cup serving*
Corn	69–87
Kidney beans	115
Lentils	106
Lima beans	95–106
Parsnips	51–70
Peas, green	57–68
Peas, split	115
Potatoes, sweet	91–146
Potatoes, white	50–59
Squash, acorn	42–57
Squash, butternut	50–70

The vegetables on *this* list are all excellent choices for a diet; each has less than 25 calories for a half-cup serving.

Asparagus	Green beans
Bean sprouts	Green pepper
Beets	Lettuce
Broccoli	Mushrooms
Brussels sprouts	Onions
Cabbage	Sauerkraut
Carrots	Spinach
Cauliflower	Squash, yellow
Celery	Squash, zucchini
Cucumber	Tomatoes
Eggplant	

Remember, though, that while some vegetables are higher in calories than others, nearly all are relatively low compared to many foods.

27. FALSE. Fiber is an essential element in a good

diet because it expedites food movement through the digestive system, but fiber itself has no magical weight loss–inducing properties. Sufficient fiber can be consumed in everyday foods without having a teaspoon of bran each day or making other drastic changes. For example, the skin of an apple has two and a half times the fiber capacity of pure bran. Fresh and frozen vegetables, fresh fruits, whole grain products, beans, and legumes are high in fiber.

28. FALSE. Some popular diets recommend severe restriction of carbohydrates, claiming that more fat is burned on this kind of diet than any other. Their rationale: when carbohydrate intake is low, the body metabolizes fat for fuel. Some of the diets allow unlimited quantities of proteins and fats. These diets can be very dangerous. Carbohydrate deprivation can cause headaches, dizziness, lethargy, and can put an added burden on the kidneys. High fat intake may contribute to heart disease. There is no evidence that this type of diet produces greater weight loss than any other diet that restricts calories to the same degree.

29. FALSE. High fat intake is sometimes a component of a low-carbohydrate diet because people like fatty foods and will, therefore, like the diet. These diets claim that fat suppresses appetite. Nutritionist Ronald M. Deutsch points out that fats leave the stomach more slowly than other food constituents and can't reach the bloodstream without passing through the small intestine, so fatty foods take longer to signal your brain that you have eaten. You can consume a great deal of fat—and consequently a great many calories—before your brain signals a halt. And since fats provide little bulk, they don't give you the nice full feeling of other foods.

Deutsch has compiled the following list to show the comparative fat content of various foods. The percentages are based on food weight, not calories. Since fat provides more than double the calories per gram of protein and carbohydrates, the percentage of calories from fat in each of the foods listed is even higher than indicated. You should also keep in mind that high-fat diets probably contribute to heart disease.

More than 90% fat:	Salad and cooking oils, fats and lard
More than 80% fat:	Butter and margarine
More than 70% fat:	Mayonnaise, macadamia nuts, pecans
More than 50% fat:	Walnuts, dried unsweetened coconut, almonds, bacon, baking chocolate
More than 30% fat:	Broiled loin steaks, spareribs, broiled pork chops, Cheddar and cream cheeses, potato chips, French dressing, chocolate candy
More than 20% fat:	Pot roast, lamb chops, frankfurters, lean ground beef, most cookies
More than 10% fat:	Most broiled fish and chicken, crabmeat, cottage cheese, beef liver, creamed soups, sherbet

30. FALSE. Laboratory studies have demonstrated that increased activity in sedentary animals actually decreases appetite. In one study with schoolchildren, scheduling activity periods *before* lunch significantly decreased food intake. Exercise may not only help you expend calories but may also curb your appetite.

31. TRUE. Vibrating belts, stationary bicycles that do the peddling for you, and other "exercise" devices at health clubs may be fun to use but lead to little energy expenditure. Some people hop on the scale when they enter a spa, use the machines, perspire away a few pounds in a sauna, and then feel as though they have accomplished something. This water loss is quickly regained.

A health club may provide you with a place and an incentive to exercise, but the type of exercise you do is more important than where you do it. Beware of questionable business practices and high-pressure salespeople at some health clubs. In the long run, a daily walk or jog may be more beneficial (and cheaper) than membership at a health club.

32. FALSE. A fat baby is probably an overfed baby. Fatness is more often associated with ill health than with good health. Fat babies are likely to become fat adolescents and then fat adults, thus relating childhood obesity to some of the most serious disorders of adulthood.

33. TRUE. The bodies of overweight children usually contain an excessive *number* of fat cells because of overfeeding. This condition, called cellular hyperplasia, is not "outgrown"; once fat cells develop, they are there for life— thus the tendency for fat children to become fat adults.

34. TRUE. When babies feed from the breast, they regulate their own intake. When they are fed from a bottle, the mother determines how much is consumed. The habit of finishing whatever is served teaches the child to ignore internal signals of hunger and places the child at the mercy of the server.

35. FALSE. A craving is more likely to develop from the *presence* of sweets in the diet than from their absence. Children fed sweets at an early age may develop a permanent "sweet tooth." The result may be a lifelong habit of eating many empty calories. Parents would be wise to introduce vegetables into an infant's diet before sweets, to develop a preference for healthy foods.

36. TRUE. Despite the current fervor for "natural" foods, once refined *or* natural sugar is digested, the result is a combination of simple sugars. The body functions the same with either type of sugar.

37. FALSE. There have been many studies on the personality characteristics of overweight people. These studies have evaluated whether overweight people are more depressed, anxious, dependent, in control of their lives, able to relate well to others, etc. Although some have found more emotional problems in overweight people than normal-weight people, *most* have found no differences. In the few cases where overweight people do show problems, it is not known whether this is a cause of the weight problem or its effect. For the most part, excess weight is not associated with any particular emotional problems.

38. TRUE. It is easy to find devices, creams, pills, lotions, and diets that promise to help you reduce in certain spots, such as thighs, hips, stomach, or midriff. However, *where* you lose weight is determined by hormones, not by a plastic sweat suit or some device that tickles your tummy. You may put weight on in certain places while a friend's bulges may be in different areas. When you lose weight, fat will be lost from all over your body. With proper exercise you can increase the muscle tone in certain areas and can speed along the general loss of fat. This will help your overall appearance; but don't expect to lose in specific areas just because you do certain exercises.

39. FALSE. If you fast (eat nothing at all), your body will use its fat stores for energy. Unfortunately, the lack of protein will lead to a loss of lean body tissue (muscle) as well as fat. In order to "spare" the body's protein, scientists have developed various protein supplements for use while fasting. A popular diet book publicized the "protein-sparing fast" idea, and millions of overweight people rushed to buy the fifty or so brands of liquid protein supplements that appeared.

The liquid protein diet has two major drawbacks. First, fasting can be very dangerous, even under the supervision of a physician (if he or she is not familiar with the associated medical complications). Second, weight gain inevitably results when the fast ends, because no new eating habits are learned to help the dieter maintain the weight loss.

Several research groups in the United States and England are continuing to study the protein-sparing modified fast, and this approach may become a useful part of a comprehensive treatment for obesity. Presently, though, such programs should be undertaken only under the strictest supervision. The popular brands of liquid protein should be avoided.

40. TRUE. Although it is easy to forget what goes on your hamburger, hot dog, or sandwich, the calories add up. A tablespoon of ketchup has more calories than a teaspoon of pure sugar, while a tablespoon of mayonnaise has more than twice the calories of a tablespoon of sugar. Commercial dressings like Russian and Thousand Island have nearly as many calories as mayonnaise. Use them in moderation (or substitute low-calorie versions); just be sure to count the calories.

41. FALSE. The body needs finite amounts of vitamins, protein, and other nutrients. Overconsumption can be as harmful as a deficiency. Vitamins A, D, E, and K are stored in the body and can become toxic at high levels. There is also little to gain from taking in more protein than you need.

42. TRUE. Despite a concerted and ambitious search, neither I nor dozens of other well-meaning scientists have been able to find any food or drink that acts as an aphrodisiac.

43. FALSE. Many people believe that there are two types of fat—regular fat and cellulite. Those visible bumps and pockets of fat on your body are called "cellulite," while the rest of the body's fat is called "fat." Many methods have been introduced for ridding the body of cellulite. However, after an extensive investigation, the American Medical Association has concluded that cellulite does not exist, that there is just one type of fat, and the devices made to dissolve cellulite are of little use.

Scoring Your Quiz

Add your correct answers and see where you rank in the official standings.

Score	Rating
38–43	*Top of the class.* You should consider an advanced degree in nutrition or in dieting science.
32–37	*Quite good.* You could do well on game shows.
23–31	*Average.* This is where most dieters score. Pay close attention to the explanations, so you won't be tripped up by diet fallacies.
11–22	*Below average.* Take a remedial dieting class.
0–10	*Below below average.* Wear a dunce hat for a day, then reread this chapter five times.

CHAPTER 16

First Aid for Food Cravings—Recipes for "Safe" Foods That Will Put You in Control

An intense craving for a particular kind of food is the undoing of many dieters. Most people respond to these yearnings either by giving in and eating extraordinary amounts of high-calorie treats, or they make themselves miserable by denying themselves the food they really want. In either case the dieter is plagued by bad feelings—guilt for a binge or dissatisfaction from denial. Your worries are over! This chapter will teach you how to cope with particular cravings.

In these pages you will find a carefully selected group of recipes, chosen to satisfy the most common cravings patients report (a desire for chocolate, or pizza, or Danish, or a milk shake, or a rich-tasting dessert, or franks, or a filling hot main dish).

When you get a yearning for a particular food, and you think a food binge is on the way, follow these simple steps:

1. Select one of the Magic Recipes that most closely fits your craving. If you need sweets, dig into a Spoonlicking Milk Shake, some Peachy-Orange Whip, or a dish of Orange Mousse. Are you hungry for chocolate? Try the Hot Chocolate Soufflé or the Hot Choco-Mocha. Would you do anything for a filling and delightful treat? Have some Raisin-

Bread Pudding or Bread-Fruit Pudding. There are many more!

2. Count your calories. You will be surprised and thrilled. You are satisfying your craving, you are eating deliciously, and you are controlling your calories!

I call these recipes "magic" because they are so tasty that you will find it hard to believe they aren't loaded with calories. You will enjoy building creative meals around them. You can serve them to guests without a qualm—they never will guess these are diet foods. You can even use these recipes to coordinate delicious menus according to the guidelines I will give you in Chapter 17.

SKINNY DIPS, DRESSINGS, SAUCES

Magic Dip

½ cup low-fat cottage
  cheese
1 tbsp. skim milk
1 green onion (scallion),
  cut up

½ small garlic clove
¼ tsp. salt
¼ tsp. paprika
1 tsp. Worcestershire sauce

Combine all ingredients in the container of a blender or food professor and blend until smooth. Use as a dip for raw vegetables, or on salads. Makes ½ cup. 14 calories per tbsp.

Roquefort Skinny-Dip

3 tbsp. skim milk
1 cup (8 oz.) low-fat cottage
  cheese
2 ounces Roquefort cheese,
  crumbled

1 tsp. Worcestershire sauce
1 tsp. lemon juice
¼ tsp. paprika

Place all ingredients in a blender and process until smooth. Serve as a dip with raw vegetables, or on salads. Makes 1½ cups. 18 calories per tbsp.

No-Oil Salad Dressing

1 cup tomato juice
1 packet chicken broth
  powder
1 tbsp. dehydrated onion
  flakes
4 tbsp. vinegar

1 tsp. mustard
2 tsp. Worcestershire sauce
⅛ tsp. garlic powder
Artificial sweetener to equal
  1 tsp. sugar

Combine all ingredients in blender container and process for a few seconds, until well mixed. Makes 1¼ cups. 5 calories per tbsp.

Tomato Sauce

2 cups tomato juice

2 tbsp. dehydrated onion
  flakes

Put tomato juice in a saucepan with the onion flakes and cook, uncovered, until reduced to 1 cup. 8 calories per tbsp.

Maple Syrup

1 tbsp. cornstarch
1 cup cold water
3 tbsp. sugar
Pinch of salt

2 tsp. maple extract
Artificial sweetener to equal
  2 tbsp. sugar

Dissolve the cornstarch in 2 tbsps. of the water, then combine with the remaining water, the sugar, and salt in a small saucepan. Cook over medium heat, stirring constantly, until the syrup thickens and bubbles. Lower the heat and simmer 1 minute. Remove from heat and stir in the maple extract and sweetener. Makes 1 cup. 12 calories per tbsp.

EYE-OPENING BREAKFAST AND LUNCH SPECIALTIES

The Toast of France

1 egg
1 tbsp. skim milk
Artificial sweetener to equal
  1 tsp. sugar

Pinch of salt
2 slices thin-sliced white
  bread
Cinnamon

Beat the egg with the milk. Add the sweetener. Soak the bread in the mixture. Brown on both sides in a nonstick frying pan. Serve sprinkled with cinnamon. 1 serving. 177 calories.

Danish Toast

¼ cup low-fat cottage
  cheese
¼ tsp. vanilla
Artificial sweetener to equal
  1 tsp. sugar

1 slice bread
Cinnamon

Combine the cottage cheese, vanilla, and artificial sweetener. Toast the bread and spread with this mixture. Sprinkle with cinnamon. Run under the broiler to heat through. Makes 1 serving. 109 calories.

Raisin-Bread Pudding

1 egg
1 slice cinnamon-raisin
  bread
¾ cup skim milk

¼ tsp. vanilla extract
Artificial sweetener to equal
  1 tsp.

Preheat the oven to 350°F. Beat the egg and put in a small baking dish with the bread, torn into small pieces, and the remaining ingredients. Bake 30 to 40 minutes, or until nicely browned. Serve hot or cold. Makes 1 serving. 210 calories.

Bread-Fruit Pudding

1 egg
½ cup crushed pineapple
(canned, no sugar added)
1 slice protein bread
¾ cup skim milk

¼ tsp. vanilla extract
Artificial sweetener to equal
1 tsp. sugar
Cinnamon

Preheat the oven to 350°F. Beat the egg and combine with the pineapple in a small baking dish. Add the bread, torn into small pieces, the milk, vanilla extract, and sweetener. Stir to combine ingredients. Sprinkle lightly with cinnamon. Bake 30 to 40 minutes, or until nicely browned. Serve hot or cold. Makes 1 serving. 258 calories.

Variation: Substitute half a small banana, sliced, for the pineapple. 234 calories.

Blueberry Muffins

2 slices whole wheat bread,
made into fine crumbs in
the blender
⅔ cup dry skim milk
powder
Artificial sweetener to equal
3 tbsp. sugar

2 tsp. baking powder
2 eggs
1 tbsp. diet margarine,
melted
1 cup blueberries, fresh or
frozen (unsweetened)

Preheat the oven to 375°F. Combine the bread crumbs, skim milk powder, sweetener, and baking powder. Beat the eggs and add with the melted margarine, stirring well to make a moist batter. Fold in the blueberries. Spoon the mixture into 6 nonstick muffin tins. Bake 20 minutes. Makes 6 muffins. 83 calories per muffin made with fresh blueberries; 106 calories per muffin made with frozen blueberries.

Cottage Eggs

3 eggs
3 oz. low-fat cottage cheese
cheese

½ tsp. salt
Dash of pepper

Beat eggs with the cottage cheese. Pour into a nonstick frying pan and cook, stirring to scramble, until set. Makes 2 servings. 156 calories per serving.

Quiche Omelet

2 eggs
1 slice (1 oz.) boiled packaged ham, minced
½ oz. Swiss cheese, grated

1 tbsp. minced onion
¼ tsp. salt
Dash of pepper

Beat the eggs with the remaining ingredients. Pour into a nonstick frying pan and cook until the bottom is set. Place under the broiler briefly, just until the top is browned and puffy. Makes 1 serving. 285 calories.

Pizza

1 slice white bread
4 oz. tomato juice, boiled
   down to half its volume
1 oz. mozzarella cheese

1 tsp. grated Parmesan
   cheese
Oregano

Toast the bread lightly. Spread with the reduced tomato juice, cover with sliced mozzarella and sprinkle with Parmesan and oregano. Broil until cheese melts and browns slightly. Makes 1 serving. 189 calories.

Pasta Chili

2 oz. lean ground beef
1 tbsp. green pepper,
   chopped
1 tsp. chopped onion
½ tsp. chili powder

3 tbsp. beef stock
3 tbsp. tomato paste
1 tbsp. water
3 oz. cooked spaghetti rings

Brown ground beef and drain off fat. Add pepper, onion, chili powder, beef stock, tomato paste, and water. Cover and simmer for 20 minutes. Add the cooked spaghetti rings and heat through. Makes 1 serving. 270 calories per serving.

SATISFYING SOUPS

Tomato-Bean Soup

1 5½-oz. can tomato juice
1 packet beef broth powder

1 8-oz. can French-style
green beans, with liquid

Combine all ingredients in a small saucepan and heat just to boiling. Makes 1 serving. 77 calories.

Clam Chowder

1 medium potato, diced
¼ cup celery, diced
1 8-oz. can chopped or
minced clams
1 cup tomato juice

1 cup chicken broth
Thyme
Hot pepper sauce
Salt
Pepper

Steam the diced potato and celery briefly in covered pan coated with Pam until just tender. Set aside. Drain the clams, reserving the juice. Combine the clam juice, tomato juice, and chicken broth. Add a pinch of thyme and a drop of hot pepper sauce. Bring to a boil and simmer five minutes, to blend flavors. Add the clams, potato, and celery and cook one more minute, to heat through. Season to taste with salt and pepper if desired. Makes 2 servings. 149 calories per serving.

Gaucho Gazpacho

4 medium tomatoes, peeled,
seeded, and cut up
½ medium cucumber,
peeled, seeded, and diced
½ raw onion, cut up
⅓ cup red wine vinegar

2 tbsp. vegetable oil
1 tsp. salt
1 garlic clove
½ tsp. pepper
Artificial sweetener to equal
1 tsp. sugar

Garnish

1 medium tomato, peeled,
  seeded, and chopped
½ medium cucumber,
  peeled, seeded, and
  chopped

1 medium green pepper,
  seeded, and diced

Place the first nine ingredients in a food processor or blender and purée. Refrigerate, covered, until thoroughly chilled, or overnight. Divide into six bowls to serve. Divide the garnish evenly between each bowl. Makes 6 servings. 70 calories per serving.

Cream-of-Anything Soup

¾ cup cooked or canned
  vegetables (peas, carrots,
  celery, zucchini, or any
  combination)
¾ cup water or vegetable
  liquid

1 packet chicken broth
  powder
1 tbsp. skim milk powder
Dash of black pepper

Heat the vegetables in the liquid with the chicken broth powder just until it reaches the boiling point. Remove from heat and pour in the blender container with the skim milk powder and pepper. Process for a few seconds, until the vegetables are puréed and the soup is creamy. Serve at once. Makes one serving. 60 to 150 calories per serving, depending on choice of vegetables.

HEARTY MAIN DISHES

Tuna and Pasta Salad

2 oz. tuna, water pack
1 oz. pasta shells
1 tomato, chopped
3 olives, chopped

3 tbsp. plain, skim milk
  yogurt
Dash of salt and pepper

Cook pasta shells in boiling water with dash of salt. Drain pasta and mix with tuna, tomato, olives, and yogurt. Season with salt and pepper and serve on lettuce. Makes 1 serving. 245 calories per serving.

Chili Burger Supreme

1 lb. lean ground beef	2 tbsp. chili sauce
1 tbsp. minced onion	2 tbsp. water
1 tsp. chili powder	

Combine beef, onion, water, chili powder, and ½ chili sauce in bowl. Mix and form 4 burgers. Put remaining chili sauce in pan and brown burgers as preferred. Makes 4 servings. 261 calories per serving.

Delta Style Chicken Jambalaya

1½ cups cooked chicken, diced	½ green pepper, chopped
	¾ cup cooked rice
1 stalk celery, chopped	¾ tsp. salt
1 cup canned tomatoes	¼ tsp. pepper
1 onion, chopped	Dash nutmeg

Combine and mix all ingredients in a casserole dish. Bake at 375° for 1 hour, stirring occasionally. Makes 3 servings. 152 calories per serving.

Veal Parmigiana

1½ lbs. veal cutlet, sliced thinly	4 tbsp. Parmesan cheese, grated
1 cup tomato sauce	⅓ cup breadcrumbs
1 egg	1 tbsp. cooking oil
1 onion, chopped	1½ oz. mozzarella cheese, sliced
1 tsp. salt	
¼ tsp. pepper	¼ tsp. basil

Mix tomato sauce, onion, and basil, and heat over low heat for 15 minutes. Beat egg, and mix with salt and pepper. Mix Parmesan cheese and breadcrumbs. Heat oil in skillet; dip veal in egg mixture, then in crumb mixture, and then brown on both sides in oil. Put veal in baking pan, cover with tomato sauce mixture, top with mozzarella cheese, and bake at 375° for 15 minutes. Makes 6 servings. 360 calories per serving.

Macaroni & Cheese Delight

3 oz. cooked macaroni
¾ oz. Cheddar cheese, shredded
1 tomato, sliced

2 oz. skim milk
1 tbsp. breadcrumbs
Dash salt

Cook macaroni, drain, and set aside. In small saucepan, heat milk and mix salt and cheese into a creamy mixture. Mix macaroni and milk-cheese sauce in a baking dish. Top with sliced tomato and sprinkle with breadcrumbs. Cover and bake at 375° for 10 minutes. Uncover and cook for 5 minutes to crisp the breadcrumbs. Makes 1 serving. 252 calories per serving.

Beef Fillet in Wine Sauce

1½ lbs. flank steak
1¼ tsp. salt
¼ tsp. pepper
½ carrot, sliced
Dash thyme

1 onion, chopped
½ tbsp. flour
½ cup beef stock
½ cup sherry
1 tbsp. parsley, chopped

Mix salt, pepper, and thyme, then rub mixture over meat. Brown meat. Add onion and carrot and brown lightly. Mix in flour gently, then mix in beef stock until mixture is blended. Roast at 350° for 15–20 minutes. Add sherry and roast additional 10–15 minutes, basting occasionally. Slice and serve on hot platter. Makes 5 servings. 319 calories per serving.

Indian Beef Pie with Curry

1 lb. lean ground beef	1 slice bread, crumbled
2 onions, chopped	2 tbsp. almonds, chopped
¼ tsp. pepper	1 tbsp. curry powder
1 tsp. salt	1 tbsp. lemon juice
2 eggs	1 tbsp. margarine
½ cup skim milk	

Melt butter and sauté onions. Mix bread, beef, onions, 1 egg, almonds, salt, pepper, lemon juice, curry powder, and put into pie pan. Beat remaining egg, mix with milk, and pour over mixture in pie pan. Bake at 350° for 1 hour. Makes 6 servings. 265 calories per serving.

Mandarin Chicken

1 frying chicken (2 pounds), sectioned	2 tbsp. margarine
11 oz. mandarin oranges, with juice	4 tbsp. lemon juice
	½ cup orange juice
¼ cup flour	2 tsp. soy sauce
2 tbsp. flour	1 tsp. Worcestershire sauce
2 tbsp. cooking oil	½ tsp. ginger
	2 tbsp. honey

Coat chicken with flour. Heat oil and margarine in skillet, then brown chicken. Mix juice from oranges with orange juice, lemon juice, soy sauce, Worcestershire sauce, honey, and ginger. Add sauce to chicken, cover, and simmer for 30 minutes. Add orange sections 5–10 minutes before chicken is done. Makes 4 servings. 335 calories per serving.

LUSCIOUS DESSERTS AND BEVERAGES

Hot Chocolate Soufflé

Butter
Flour
2 egg whites
3 tbsp. unsweetened cocoa
    powder

3 tbsp. sugar
¼ tsp. cinnamon
¼ tsp. vanilla extract
¼ tsp. rum extract

Preheat the oven to 350°F. Prepare two custard cups by buttering sparingly. Sprinkle with flour and shake out the excess. Beat two egg whites until they are stiff enough to hold peaks. Combine the cocoa, sugar, and cinnamon and fold gently into the egg whites. Add the vanilla and rum extracts. Spoon the soufflé mixture into the two custard cups. Set the cups into a baking dish and pour boiling water into the dish until it reaches about three quarters of the way up the outside of the custard cups. Bake 30 minutes. Serve warm. Makes 2 servings. 125 calories per serving.

Stop-and-Go Parfait

1 envelope (4-serving size)
    strawberry-flavored low-
    calorie gelatin dessert
1 cup boiling water
5 ice cubes

1 envelope (4-serving size)
    lime-flavored low-calorie
    gelatin dessert
1 cup boiling water
5 ice cubes

Dissolve the strawberry gelatin in one cup of boiling water. Add the ice cubes and stir until thickened, about 5 minutes. Do the same with the lime gelatin. Divide half of the thickened strawberry gelatin between 4 parfait glasses. Place in the freezer for 9 minutes, to set. Divide half of the lime gelatin between the 4 glasses and return to the freezer for 9 minutes, until the green "stripes" set. Repeat with the remaining red and green gelatin. Chill until firm. Serves 4. 20 calories per serving.

Orange Mousse

¾ cup boiling water
2 envelopes (2 tbsp.)
  unflavored gelatin
6-oz. can frozen orange juice
  concentrate, undiluted

1 tsp. vanilla extract
Artificial sweetener to equal
  4 tsp. sugar
2 cups skim milk

Put the water and gelatin in a blender and process to dissolve the gelatin. Add the remaining ingredients and process at high speed for a few seconds. Pour into a bowl or individual serving dishes. Refrigerate until firm, about 2 hours, or overnight. Makes 10 servings. 60 calories per serving.

Peachy-Orange Whip

1 envelope (4-serving size)
  orange-flavored low-
  calorie gelatin dessert
½ cup boiling water

5 ice cubes
4 peach halves (canned, no
  sugar added)

Dissolve the gelatin dessert in the boiling water. Add the ice cubes and stir until thickened, about 5 minutes. Remove any unmelted ice and whip until thick and fluffy. Divide half of the gelatin between 4 parfait glasses. Top each with a peach half, sliced. When slightly set spoon the rest of the gelatin over the peach slices in each glass. Makes 4 servings. 35 calories per serving.

Dreamy Whipped Topping

⅓ cup skim milk powder
⅓ cup ice water
2 tsp. lemon juice

1 tsp. vanilla extract
Artificial sweetener to equal
  3 tbsp. sugar

Combine all ingredients in a bowl and beat 10 minutes at top speed with an electric mixer, until the mixture is stiff and stands in peaks. Serve immediately. If left to stand, the topping will liquefy; however, you can rewhip to fluff it up again. Makes 4 servings, the equivalent of ¼ cup of skim milk each. 25 calories per serving.

Hot Choco-Mocha

¾ cup skim milk
1 tsp. instant coffee
1 tsp. vanilla extract
1 tsp. chocolate extract

Artificial sweetener to equal
   1 tsp. sugar
Nutmeg

Heat the milk in a saucepan with the instant coffee, vanilla and chocolate extracts, and the sweetener. When hot, pour into a blender and process for a few seconds, just until frothy. Pour into a mug and sprinkle with nutmeg. Makes 1 serving. 80 calories.

Piña Colada

6 oz. skim milk
¼ cup crushed pineapple,
   with juice
1 tbsp. shredded unsweet-
   ened coconut

¼ tsp. rum extract
½ tsp. vanilla extract
Artificial sweetener to equal
   2 tsp. sugar
2 ice cubes

Combine all ingredients except ice cubes in a blender. Process at high speed until thick and smooth, adding one ice cube at a time while the motor is running. Makes 1 serving. 140 calories.

Rum Toddy

4 oz. skim milk
½ tsp. rum extract

¼ tsp. vanilla extract
Nutmeg

Heat the milk to just below the boiling point. Remove from heat and season with the rum and vanilla extracts. Pour into a punch cup. Sprinkle wtih nutmeg. Makes 1 serving. 48 calories.

Café au Lait

4 oz. skim milk
4 oz. black coffee
Artificial sweetener to equal
  ½ tsp. sugar (or to taste)

Cinnamon stick
Dreamy Whipped Topping
  (see above) (optional)

Combine the milk and coffee in a small saucepan and heat to just below the boiling point. Pour into a mug, sweeten, and stir with a cinnamon stick. Makes 1 serving. 40 calories. If desired, fluff on one serving of Dreamy Whipped Topping: the calories will now total 65.

Spoon-Licking Milk Shakes

Coffee Milk Shake
6 oz. skim milk
1 tsp. powered coffee
  (regular or decaffeinated)
½ tsp. vanilla extract

Artificial sweetener to equal
  1 tsp. sugar (or to taste)
2 ice cubes

Put all ingredients except ice cubes in a blender. Process at high speed until thick and smooth, adding one ice cube at a time while the motor is running. Makes 1 serving. 70 calories.

Maple Milk Shake
6 oz. skim milk
½ tsp. maple extract
½ tsp. vanilla extract

Artificial sweetener to equal
  1 tsp. sugar (or to taste)
2 ice cubes

Prepare as above. Makes 1 serving. 70 calories.

Strawberry Milk Shake
6 oz. skim milk
5 fresh strawberries
½ tsp. vanilla extract
¼ tsp. almond extract

Artificial sweetener to equal
  1 tsp. sugar (or to taste)
2 ice cubes

Prepare as above. Makes 1 serving. 85 calories.

Variations: Use a third of a banana (34 calories) and coco-nut extract instead of the strawberries and almond extract. Or use ¼ cup fresh blueberries (43 calories) . . . a fresh peach (38 calories) . . . whatever fruit you most enjoy.

CHAPTER 17

Delicious Menus for Your Lifestyle: More Than One Hundred Meals for Real-World Eating

Here are 124 "safe" menus that are for eating in the *real* world. They contain not only conventional foods, but fast foods for eating on the run, and frozen convenience foods for when you are in a hurry at home. This menu plan provides maximum flexibility for *your* eating lifestyle, yet its boundaries provide the structure you will need at certain times. Many diets forbid the foods you really crave. Still others are so unstructured that you don't have real assistance in times of need. The menus in this chapter remedy each of these problems.

There are five reasons why these menus will soothe your taste buds and trim your waist:

1. *You Choose from a Month's Worth of Breakfasts, Lunches, Dinners, and Snacks*

There are 31 breakfasts, 31 lunches, and the same number of dinners and snacks. You can eat for an entire month just using these menus, and with the substitutions you are allowed, you will have endless choices of delicious foods. On any given day you can choose from any of the 124 menus. You are *not* required to eat a specific meal any day, so you will be eating foods you enjoy. Here's how it works.

For any meal select a menu that contains foods you like. The calories for each menu are listed, so you can make prudent choices according to your own eating plan. Let's say, for example, that you arrive home one evening and you have 350–400 calories remaining before you reach your calorie total for the day. You can choose from many delicious dinners under 400 calories and still stay within your daily total. There are many meals for days when you have 600 or more calories remaining for the day. The menus are ranked from the least number of calories to the most, so you can easily find one that fits your pattern for the day.

2. *These Are Real-World Menus*

One recent study indicated that the average American eats fewer than 50 percent of his meals at home. Therefore, it is important to have an eating strategy for meals away from home as well as for meals at home. These menus take into account the realities of today's world. You can now have meal plans that include fast foods, frozen foods, and the traditional basic foods. These will help you master *any* situation.

3. *The Menus Fit YOUR Eating Style*

Many dieters eat small breakfasts, small lunches, and large dinners. Others have large lunches but eat very little at other meals. Your eating style may fit one of many patterns, and your pattern may not be the same every day. How, then, can you adhere to a rigid meal plan that dictates exactly what to eat day after day? The answer is simple— you can't.

These menus can fit your lifestyle. If you are a lunch person, choose a big lunch. If you feel like a hearty dinner, you will have many choices. Since the menus are ordered according to calories, you can pick a meal according to your specifications and still maintain your calorie level for the day. You may even want to experiment with meals of different sizes to see which pattern is easiest for you to follow.

4. *You Are Free to Substitute Your Favorite Foods*

These menus are designed to provide *possibilities* for meals. In any menu, you may like some of the foods and dislike others. Be creative and substitute foods you like the most and foods you have available. If you find flounder on sale, use flounder. Use leftovers as substitutes, or use the Magic Recipes in Chapter 16.

Your choices for substitutes are unlimited. The Appendixes of this book contain three calorie guides unequaled in any existing weight-loss book—a Basic Foods Guide, a Fast-Foods Guide, and a Frozen Convenience Foods Guide. Use these to substitute creatively. Remember the nutrition guidelines in Chapter 4 as you plan your meals, and be certain to remember your calorie limits for the day.

Here are some examples for substitutes:

Item from Original Menu		*Substitutes*	
Food	*Calories*	*Food*	*Calories*
Egg salad sandwich	280	Corned beef sandwich	304
		Bacon, lettuce, tomato sandwich	280
		Bologna sandwich	248
		Chicken salad sandwich	245
6 oz. lean, trimmed round steak	321	Chicken fricassee	368
		Fried chicken, 2 breasts	320
		Broiled ham, 4 oz.	266
		Polish sausage	240

Which fast-food restaurants are most convenient for you?

Item from Original Menu		*Substitutes*	
Food	*Calories*	*Food*	*Calories*
Arthur Treacher's Shrimp	381	Arby's Roast Beef	350
		Burger Chef Double Cheeseburger	430
		Kentucky Fried Chicken, 1 thigh	275
		Pizza Hut, ½ 10 in. pepperoni pizza	430

What is your preference in frozen foods?

Birds Eye Carrots w/ Brown Sugar Glaze	80	Birds Eye Green Peas w/ Sliced Mushrooms	70
		Green Giant Asparagus w/ Butter Sauce	90
		LaChoy Beef Chow Mein	97
		Stokely Chuckwagon Corn	90

5. *You Have the Right Balance between Structure and Flexibility*

I don't expect or intend for you to use these menus all of the time. You are the best judge of when you need specific meal plans.

These menus are unique because of the structure they provide. You can use them to make eating a pleasant experience and vary them by substituting from the foods you most enjoy.

BREAKFASTS FOR A MONTH

		Calories				*Calories*
1.	tangerine	39		6.	1 cup corn flakes	97
	1 cup Special K				1 fresh peach,	
	cereal	70			sliced	38
	½ cup skim milk	40			½ cup skim milk	40
		149			black coffee	5
						180

		Calories				*Calories*
2.	½ cup fresh straw-			7.	½ grapefruit	40
	berries and ⅓				poached egg	82
	small banana,				½ English muffin	70
	sliced	53			1 tsp. diet	
	1 cup puffed rice				margarine	17
	cereal	60				209
	½ cup skim milk	40				
		153				

				8.	1 cup puffed rice	
3.	½ cup tomato				cereal	50
	juice	23			½ banana, sliced	51
	¾ cup oatmeal	98			½ cup skim milk	40
	½ cup skim milk	40			1 slice whole wheat	
		161			bread	56
					1 tsp. diet	
					margarine	17
						214

				9.	tangerine	39
4.	½ cup tomato				1 cup raisin bran	
	juice	23			flakes	144
	1 egg, soft-boiled	82			½ cup skim milk	40
	2 pieces Melba					223
	toast	50				
	1 tsp. cream cheese	19				
		174				

				10.	½ cantaloupe	60
5.	1 oz. shredded				bagel (2 oz.)	165
	wheat	85			1 tsp. cream cheese	17
	½ banana	51				242
	½ cup skim milk	40				
		176				

	Calories			Calories
11. ½ cup orange juice	53		2 tbsp. Maple Syrup*	36
soft-boiled egg	82			271
bran muffin	104			
1 tsp. diet margarine	17	16.	1 orange	64
	256		Raisin-Bread Pudding*	210
				274
12. ½ cup tomato juice	23			
Bread-Fruit Pudding*	234	17.	½ cup tomato juice	23
	257		1 poached egg	82
			2 slices bacon	86
			½ English muffin	70
13. ½ cup apricot nectar	72		1 tsp. diet margarine	17
Danish Toast*	109			278
poached egg	82			
	263	18.	1 cup diced cantaloupe	70
			2 pieces toast	158
14. bagel (approx. 2 oz.)	165		1 tsp. jam	54
1 oz. creamed cottage cheese	30			282
1 oz. smoked salmon	50	19.	6 oz. orange juice	77
coffee with half & half	25		2 Blueberry Muffins*	212
	270			289
15. ¼ cantaloupe filled with ½ cup strawberries	58	20.	½ grapefruit	40
The Toast of France*	177		English muffin topped with 1 oz. melted Cheddar cheese	251
				291

* Recipes can be found in Chapter 16.

Calories   *Calories*

21. 6 oz. orange juice   80
  Cottage Eggs*   156
  1 slice whole wheat
   bread   56
  1 tsp. jam   <u>18</u>
       310

22. ½ grapefruit   40
  Danish Toast*   109
  2 poached eggs   <u>162</u>
       311

23. 5 oz. orange juice   67
  English muffin
   topped with
   1 oz. melted
   Cheddar cheese   <u>251</u>
       318

24. ½ grapefruit   40
  poached egg   82
  2 Blueberry
   Muffins*   212
  1 tsp. diet
   margarine   <u>17</u>
       351

25. McDonald's Egg
  McMuffin   350
  black coffee   <u>5</u>
       355

26. 1 cup bran flakes   130
  ½ cup sliced
   strawberries   28
  ½ cup skim milk   40

English muffin   140
1 tsp. diet
 margarine   <u>17</u>
       355

27. ½ cup tomato
  juice   23
  4 small buttermilk
   pancakes   244
  2 tbsp. Maple
   Syrup*   28
  2 strips of bacon   <u>86</u>
       381

28. 1 cup fresh
  grapefruit &
  orange sections   91
  1 cup cooked cream
   of wheat   130
  ½ cup skim milk   40
  bran muffin   104
  1 tsp. diet
   margarine   <u>17</u>
       382

29. 2 brown & serve
  sausage links   144
  2 large scrambled
   eggs   222
  ½ cup orange
   juice   <u>53</u>
       419

30. 4 small buttermilk
  pancakes   244

* Recipes can be found in Chapter 16.

	Calories			Calories
3 tbsp. Maple Syrup*	42	31.	McDonald's Hot Cakes with Butter and Syrup	470
2 brown & serve sausage links	144		coffee with milk	15
	430			485

LUNCHES FOR A MONTH

	Calories			Calories
1. chicken noodle soup, 1 cup	62	5. 1 cup minestrone	105
cucumber spears	15	Pizza*	189
tomato wedges	27		294
2 tbsp. Roquefort Skinny-Dip*	36		
	140	6. 1 cup minestrone	105
		Buitoni Lasagna w/Meat Sauce	168
2. turkey noodle soup, 1 cup	79	salad (1 cup lettuce, 3 radishes, ½ cucumber)	21
sliced tomato	27	2 tbsp. No-Oil Salad Dressing*	10
1 tbsp. Magic Dip*	14		304
Hot Choco-Mocha*	80		
	200	7. McDonald's Cheeseburger	306
		diet soda	0
3. egg-tomato sandwich	150		306
apple	96		
	246	8. egg salad sandwich on white bread	280
		½ cup coleslaw	30
4. 1 cup unflavored skim milk yogurt	123		310
1 grated apple	96	9. ½ cup uncreamed cottage cheese	98
1 grated carrot	30	½ cup canned water-pack grapefruit sections	37
1 tsp. honey	22		
	271		

* Recipes can be found in Chapter 16.

		Calories
	1 apple	96
	10 grapes	34
	1 tbsp. chopped walnuts	50
		315
10.	1 cup firm-cooked spaghetti	192
	½ cup clams with liquid	50
	6 artichoke hearts with 2 tbsp. diet Italian dressing	60
	Stop-and-Go Parfait*	20
		322
11.	Arthur Treacher's Krunch Pups	203
	Cole Slaw	123
		326
12.	Pasta Chilli*	270
	4 medium asparagus spears	12
	1 slice protein bread	45
		327
13.	White Castle Hamburger	165
	½ order Onion Rings	171
		336
14.	1 cup firm-cooked spaghetti	192

		Calories
	½ cup Tomato Sauce*	64
	½ cup green beans	16
	1 cup celery and carrot sticks	40
	2 tbsp. Roquefort Skinny-Dip*	36
		348
15.	Tuna & Pasta Salad*	245
	bran muffin	104
		349
16.	1 cup firm-cooked spaghetti	192
	½ cup Tomato Sauce*	64
	1 tbsp. grated Parmesan cheese	29
	1 cup mixed greens	20
	3 tbsp. Roquefort Skinny-Dip*	54
		359
17.	peanut butter sandwich	
	1 tbsp. peanut butter	94
	2 slices whole wheat bread	112
	1 cup skim milk	80
	apple	96
		382
18.	Stouffer Frozen Cheese Pizza	330

* Recipes can be found in Chapter 16.

Calories   *Calories*

	salad (1 cup let-tuce, 1 scallion, 5 radishes)	22
	2 tbsp. Roquefort Skinny-Dip*	36
		388
19.	ham and cheese sandwich	336
	6 oz. skim milk	60
		396
20.	Pizza Hut Thin & Crispy Pepperoni (½ 10″ Pizza	430
	diet soda	0
		430
21.	Taco Bell Tostada	206
	Pintos 'N Cheese	231
		437
22.	Gaucho Gazpacho*	70
	4 oz. broiled hamburger	324
	1 slice protein bread	45
		439
23.	bacon, lettuce, and tomato sandwich on white bread	280
	1 cup skim milk	80
	apple	96
		456

24.	bologna and cheese sandwich	355
	1 dill pickle	7
	apple	96
		458
25.	knockwurst, 2 4-inch links	278
	1 oz. Gouda cheese	108
	1 cup skim milk	80
		466
26.	Clam Chowder*	149
	tuna salad sandwich	280
	1 cup celery & carrot sticks	40
		469
27.	ham & cheese sandwich	336
	fig bar	50
	pear	86
		472
28.	Burger King Whaler	486
	Iced Tea	0
		486
29.	Burger Chef Cheeseburger	300
	French Fried Potatoes	190
		490

* Recipes can be found in Chapter 16.

	Calories		*Calories*
30. Tomato-Bean		31. Arby's Roast Beef	350
Soup*	77	Baskin-Robbins	
Morton Frozen		Chocolate Fudge	
Beef Pie	390	Ice Cream (1	
Orange Mousse*	60	scoop)	178
	527		528

DINNERS FOR A MONTH

	Calories		*Calories*
1. La Choy Chicken		5. Indian Beef Pie	
Chow Mein	97	with Curry*	265
La Choy Shrimp		½ cup green	
Egg Roll	108	beans	16
⅓ cup instant rice	60	sliced cucumber	15
	265	1 tbsp. Roquefort	
		Skinny-Dip*	18
2. Stouffer Tuna			314
Noodle Cas-			
serole	200	6. Delta Style	
1 cup broccoli	48	Chicken	
Peachy-Orange		Jambalaya*	152
Whip*	35	½ cup zucchini	22
	283	½ med. baked	
		potato	73
3. Macaroni & Cheese		1 tbsp. sour cream	29
Delight*	252	Orange Mousse*	60
1 cup carrots	48		336
	300		
		7. 4 oz. broiled	
4. Chili Burger		chicken	154
Supreme*	261	½ cup instant rice	90
sliced tomato	27	1 cup asparagus	
1 tbsp. Magic Dip*	14	tips	94
	302		338

* Recipes can be found in Chapter 16.

		Calories			*Calories*

8. Tuna & Pasta
   Salah* — 245
   ½ cup green beans — 16
   2 tangerines — 78
   339

9. 8 oz. baked sole — 180
   Birds Eye Frozen
   Green Beans &
   Pearl Onions — 35
   Birds Eye Carrots
   with Brown
   Sugar Glaze — 80
   Birds Eye Shredded
   Hash Browns — 60
   355

10. broiled chicken
    (6 oz.) — 231
    parsley-boiled
    potato — 106
    tomato, cucumber,
    & red onion
    salad — 45
    382

11. 1 cup beef broth — 31
    chicken liver kabobs
    (4 oz. chicken
    livers, 4 cherry
    tomatoes, ½
    onion, ½ green
    pepper) — 239
    ½ cup brown rice — 116
    386

12. Indian Beef Pie
    with Curry* — 265

salad (1 cup let-
tuce, 1 scallion,
5 radishes) — 22
2 tbsp. diet blue
cheese dressing — 24
Green Giant Boil-
in-Bag Spinach
in Butter Sauce — 90
401

13. Mrs. Paul's Fried
    Fish Fillets — 220
    ½ cup instant rice — 90
    1 cup French-style
    green beans — 34
    1 slice garlic bread
    (made with 1
    piece French
    bread, ½ pat
    butter) — 62
    406

14. 4 oz. broiled
    chicken — 154
    ½ cup instant rice — 90
    1 cup cauliflower — 32
    1 cup carrots — 48
    1 brown & serve
    roll — 84
    408

15. Beef Fillet in Wine
    Sauce* — 319
    ½ cup carrots — 24
    salad (1 cup let-
    tuce, 1 tomato) — 37

* Recipes can be found in Chapter 16.

	Calories
2 tbsp. diet French dressing	30
	410

16. Veal Parmigiana* 360
    1 cup broccoli 48
    1 sliced tomato 27
    —
    435

17. Veal Parmigiana* 360
    ⅓ cup instant rice 60
    ½ cup carrots 24
    Stop-and-Go Parfait* 20
    —
    464

18. 4 oz. leg of lamb, lean 211
    3 oz. Ore-Ida Tater Tots 160
    3.3 oz. Birds Eye Baby Brussels Sprouts 35
    Orange Mousse* with Whipped Topping* 85
    —
    491

19. Chili Burger Supreme* 261
    ½ cup instant rice 90
    1 cup broccoli 48
    ½ sliced cucumber 8
    2 tbsp. No-Oil Salad Dressing* 10
    1 slice French bread 44

	Calories
1 pat butter	36
	497

20. broiled chicken, 6 oz. 231
    1 cup broccoli 48
    tomato, cucumber, & red onion salad 45
    pear 86
    1 oz. Gorgonzola cheese 112
    —
    522

21. Mandarin Chicken* 335
    ⅓ cup instant rice 60
    Green Giant Boil-in-Bag Chinese Style Vegetables 130
    —
    525

22. Long John Silver Shrimp with Batter 269
    Hush Puppies 134
    Cole Slaw 133
    —
    536

23. Swanson Frozen Chicken Pie 450
    ½ cup green beans 16
    Maple Milk Shake* 70
    —
    536

24. Beef Fillet in Wine Sauce* 319
    ½ cup noodles 100

* Recipes can be found in Chapter 16.

	Calories
1 cup broccoli	48
Orange Mousse*	
with Whipped	
Topping*	85
	552

25. Banquet Beef En-
    chilada — 479
    pear — 86
    565

26. 6 oz. lean, trimmed
    round steak — 321
    baked potato — 145
    1 tbsp. sour cream — 29
    1 tsp. chives — 1
    1 cup green beans — 43
    Stop-and-Go Par-
    fait* with
    Whipped Top-
    ping* — 45
    584

27. 4 oz. lean lamb
    w/mint sauce — 300
    ¾ cup brown rice — 174
    1 cup zucchini — 22
    1 cup carrots — 48
    tomato & onion
    salad — 55
    599

28. 4 oz. lean, trimmed
    sirloin steak — 235

	Calories
1 cup mashed pota-	
toes w/milk	137
1 cup broccoli	48
sliced cucumber	15
2 tbsp. No-Oil	
Salad Dressing*	10
1 chocolate devil's	
food cupcake,	
iced	162
	607

29. ¼ cantaloupe — 30
    Swanson Fried
    Chicken TV
    Dinner — 570
    Stop-and-Go Par-
    fait* — 20
    620

30. Mandarin
    Chicken* — 335
    ⅓ cup instant rice — 60
    ½ cup lima beans — 95
    1 cup salad greens — 10
    2 tbsp. No-Oil
    Salad Dressing* — 10
    Hot Chocolate
    Soufflé* — 125
    635

31. Arthur Treacher's
    Shrimp — 381
    Chips — 276
    657

* Recipes can be found in Chapter 16.

SNACKS FOR A MONTH

		Calories
1.	1 cup unbuttered popcorn	23
2.	celery & carrot sticks	37
3.	tangerine	39
4.	1 slice fresh pineapple	44
5.	1 cup raw radishes, celery, and zucchini	18
	3 tbsp. Magic Dip*	42
		60
6.	Maple Milk Shake*	70
7.	Coffee Milk Shake*	70
8.	1 cup beef broth	31
	3 pieces melba toast	45
		76
9.	Tomato-Bean Soup*	77
10.	2 peaches	78
11.	1 cup strawberries	55
	Whipped Topping*	25
		80
12.	Hot Choco-Mocha*	80

		Calories
13.	1 cup fresh strawberries with ¼ cup orange juice	82
14.	1 cup mixed raw vegetables (zucchini, cauliflower, carrot)	33
	3 tbsp. Roquefort Skinny-Dip*	54
		87
15.	1 cup water-pack fruit cocktail	91
16.	1 cup tomato juice	46
	5 Wheat Thins	50
		96
17.	Café au Lait*	40
	2 gingersnaps	60
		100
18.	Peachy Orange Whip* with Whipped Topping*	60
	1 chocolate chip cookie	50
		110
19.	Orange Sherbet (¼ pint)	114
20.	½ cup strawberry yogurt	130

* Recipes can be found in Chapter 16.

		Calories			*Calories*
21.	1 cup skim milk	80	27.	Piña Colada*	140
	2 graham crackers	60		1 graham cracker	30
		140			170
22.	Piña Colada*	140	28.	bagel (2 oz.)	165
				1 tsp. cream	
23.	1 banana, sliced	101		cheese	17
	2 tbsp. half & half	40			182
		141			
			29.	1 cup beef noodle	
24.	1 cup split pea			soup	67
	soup	146		1 slice pumper-	
				nickel	80
25.	pound cake	142		pat of butter	36
	black coffee	5			183
		147			
			30.	1 cup unsweetened	
26.	½ cantaloupe	60		apple sauce	100
	½ cup uncreamed			3 gingersnaps	90
	cottage cheese	98			190
		158	31.	raspberry yogurt	260

* Recipes can be found in Chapter 16.

CHAPTER **18**

The Last Word

Now that you are finishing this book, we can start planning for the future. The entire program is designed to culminate at this point—the very point where you take complete command of your weight. It will be in the years ahead that you prove how effective Partnership Dieting really is. Very few programs will get you this far, and no other program will create a plan for you to control your weight permanently. You and your partner can make this program work. Remember what I said on the first page of this book—Together Is Better!

Dieters get most anxious at the *end* of diet programs. This happens for a good reason—most diet programs do not teach the dieter to deal with the weeks, months, and years that follow the diet. Robin experienced this many times: "I have lost weight in the past, but I always gain it back. I get depressed when I regain the weight and I feel like a complete failure. I am scared to death that this will happen again." Are Robin's feelings like yours?

The Partnership Program is different from any other diet. The strength of the Partnership Program lies in its long-term effectiveness. My research and that of others has shown that Partnership Dieting leads to improved *maintenance* of weight loss. How does this work?

First, working with your partner can make this the most successful diet you have ever tried. There will be times when your motivation will decline—this happens to all dieters. With Partnership Dieting your partner can bail you out during difficult times. In essence, you have a double dose of motivation—yours and your partner's. Since dieting is a long-term enterprise, you may get lonely having to bear the burden of a weight problem. Your partner's interest and support will give you just the boost you need during these lonely periods. Dieters often feel that there is no reward for the constant vigilance that is required for sustained weight loss. Your partner can remedy this absence of support by encouraging your efforts.

Partnership Dieting will be effective for *maintaining* weight loss because you have developed behaviors that are becoming permanent eating habits. As these techniques become part of your daily repertoire of activities, you will be able to lose weight with less and less effort. These behaviors will replace the old habits that led to your weight gain. This fact sets the Partnership plan apart from the diets that emphasize only *what* you eat, not *how* to eat.

If you were on a conventional diet, you would be saying, "How can I live with these foods I have to eat, and how can I go without the foods I love?" I want you to eat the foods you love most, and I do not want to force you to eat foods you dislike. This is necessary if you are to live with any program for more than a brief time. You will enjoy your eating *more* as a result of the program. You can live with a program if you can eat deliciously and lose weight at the same time.

Making the Program Work

You have all the tools you need to build a successful and lasting weight-loss program. The techniques you have used during this program will help you deal with dieting more effectively. By using the procedures you have learned, you will take control over the factors that controlled you.

Several things probably will happen to you as time goes

on. Not all dieters go through these stages, but most do. First, there will be times when it seems you have lost control of your weight. You will begin reverting to some of your old eating habits, and you may begin to gain weight. *This* is not a crisis. However, your *reaction* to such an event can turn it into a crisis. Would you respond like this dieter? "I really have blown it now. After all the work I put in, I can't even keep the weight off. This proves that I am a failure and that I will never be able to keep my weight down." These self-defeating attitudes can ruin your program unless you recognize their presence and counter them with your new methods of coping.

The attitude techniques described in Chapter 10 will immunize you against attacks of self-defeating emotions. Practice these techniques and be prepared for brief lapses. Right now I want you to repeat to yourself, "I know there will be times when I won't do as well as I should. I will be prepared for these times so I won't give up and feel terrible. I can get back to the program even if I have overeaten and if I have gained weight." With this attitude, you will not be sidetracked by the inevitable setbacks that everyone experiences.

This book should be a permanent resource for you. You have learned the principles of the program, and you can use the techniques for lasting weight loss. Use the book when you need booster shots. The book will remind you about the best ways to analyze and solve your dieting problems. The crisis intervention chapters (13 and 14) will be especially valuable because they deal with the difficult situations that you are bound to encounter.

Start planning right now for the next stages of your program. Use the blank Diet Diary page provided in Chapter 5 to maintain your careful monitoring of calories. Some dieters find a high correlation between their ability to control their weight and the dedication with which they complete the Diet Diary. In addition, use the blank Daily Log from Chapter 12 to make your Permanent Daily Log. This can be used indefinitely. It will remind you of the most important behaviors for your program and will provide you with an indication of your success.

Partner, the end of the sixteen weeks does not signal the end of your support and encouragement. Dieting is not like an infection that is treated and then forgotten. Dieting requires constant attention, from both you and the dieter. Your efforts can become less intense as times goes on, as the dieter develops new habits that will insure the maintenance of weight loss. However, your *most* important impact can come during the upcoming months and years.

Partner, there will be times when the dieter's motivation will fade, when the dieter has eating binges, and when the dieter will gain weight. These points are *critical*. If you and the dieter give up hope in a fit of despair, you will be placing a psychological obstacle in your path to success. This book is a permanent resource for you. Use the crisis intervention chapters (13 and 14) to help the dieter through difficult situations. You are in command of a program that can boost the dieter through any situation!

Dieter and Partner, you have just completed one of the most comprehensive programs for weight control ever developed. This is the first program ever to use the Partnership approach. For these two reasons I am confident that you can lose weight and keep it off. You have learned dozens of behavioral techniques, and you have learned many ways to increase your physical activity. You know how important your attitudes and emotions can be, and you have learned how to cope with the depressing moments every dieter faces. You now can avoid the failure factors that doom other diets to poor results. In other words, you have learned everything that it takes to be a thin person! You now can be the master of your own destiny!

GOOD LUCK!!

PART 5

Appendixes: The Calorie Guide Handbook

In these pages you will find the most comprehensive guide to calories that ever has been assembled! It covers all the basic foods and beverages, the nation's most popular fast foods, and the frozen convenience foods you find in your supermarket.

The Basic Foods Calorie Guide

These values are based on data published in the U.S. Department of Agriculture Handbook No. 465, and by the Smith, Kline, and French Laboratories.

Calories are listed for average serving sizes whenever possible. You may wish to convert some measurements to others to simplify matters. For example, some beverages are listed in fluid ounces while others are listed in cups. Several measurement equivalents are presented below to help with this task.

Measurement Equivalents
1 cup = 8 fluid ounces
1 cup = ½ pint
1 cup = 16 tablespoons
2 tablespoons = 1 fluid ounce
1 tablespoon = 3 teaspoons
1 quart = 4 cups
1 pound = 16 ounces

CALORIE VALUES FOR FOODS AND BEVERAGES

Food	*Calories*
"A"	
Abalone, canned, 4 oz.	91
Acerola, 10 fruits	23
Albacore, (see tuna)	
Alcoholic beverages (see beverages)	
Ale (see beverages)	

Food	*Calories*
Almonds	
dried, in shell, 1 cup	187
dried, in shell, 10 nuts	60
shelled, whole, 1 cup	849
chopped, 1 cup	777
roasted (in oil), 1 cup	984
roasted (in oil), 1 ounce (app. 22 nuts)	178
Anchovy	
drained from can, 1⅗ oz.	79
5 medium fillets	35
Apples	
1 raw with skin, 3″ diam. (app. 2½ per pound)	96
1 raw, peeled, 3″ diam. (app. 2½ per pound)	85
dehydrated, sulfured, 1 cup	353
1 baked, with 2 tbsp. sugar	172
frozen, sweetened, sliced ½ cup	93
Apple Brown Betty, 1 cup	325
Apple butter, 1 tbsp.	33
Apple drink, canned commercial brand, 4 oz.	58
Apple juice, 1 cup	117
Apple Sauce	
unsweetened, 1 cup	100
sweetened, 1 cup	232
Apricots	
raw, 3 medium	55
raw, halves, 1 cup	79
canned, water pack, 1 cup	93
canned, syrup pack, 1 cup	222
dried, uncooked, 1 cup	338
dried, cooked, unsweetened, 1 cup	213
dried, cooked, sweetened, 1 cup	329
Apricot nectar, 1 cup	143
Artichoke, globe, cooked, 1 medium	53
Artichoke hearts, frozen, 3 hearts	22
Asparagus	
raw spears, 1 cup	35
raw, 5–6 spears	26
cooked spears, 4 medium	12

Food	*Calories*
canned spears, 1 cup	94
frozen, cuts and tips, boiled, 1 cup	40
Avocados	
California, 1 medium	378
California, cubed, 1 cup	257
Florida, 1 medium	389
Florida, cubed, 1 cup	192

"B"

Bacon	
raw, sliced, 1 pound	3,016
cooked, 2 medium slices	86
Canadian, cooked, 1 slice	58
Bagel, 1 water	55
Baking powder, 1 tbsp.	14
Bamboo shoots, 1 cup	40
Bananas	
raw, 1 medium	101
raw, sliced, 1 cup	128
raw, mashed, 1 cup	191
dehydrated (banana flakes), 1 ounce	96
Barbecue sauce, 1 cup	228
Barley, pearl, scotched, 1 tbsp.	44
Bass	
black sea, baked, stuffed, 1 oz.	73
striped, oven fried, 1 oz.	56
Beans	
great northern, raw, 1 cup	612
great northern, cooked, 1 cup	212
navy (pea), cooked, 1 cup	224
white, canned, with pork & tomato sauce, 1 cup	311
white, canned, with pork & sweet sauce, 1 cup	383
kidney, raw, 1 cup	635
kidney, cooked, 1 cup	218
kidney, canned, 1 cup	230
pinto, raw, 1 cup	663
lima, raw, 1 cup	191
lima, cooked, 1 cup	189

Food	Calories
lima, canned, 1 cup	176
lima, frozen, cooked, 1 cup	168
green, raw, 1 cup	35
green, cooked, 1 cup	31
green, canned, 1 cup	43
green, frozen, cooked, 1 cup	34
green, French style, cooked, 1 cup	34
yellow (wax), cooked, 1 cup	28
yellow (wax), canned, 1 cup	45
yellow (wax), frozen, cooked, 1 cup	36
Bean sprouts, mung, raw, 1 cup	20
Bean sprouts, soy, raw, 1 cup	45
Beans and frankfurters, 1 cup	367
Beechnuts, shelled, 1 lb.	2,576
Beef	
brisket, lean & fat, braised, 4 oz	470
brisket, lean, trimmed of fat, braised, 4 oz.	253
chuck, arm, lean & fat, pot roasted, 4 oz.	329
chuck, arm, lean, trimmed of fat, pot roasted, 4 oz.	220
chuck, rib, lean & fat, pot roasted, 4 oz.	487
chuck, rib, lean, trimmed of fat, pot roasted, 4 oz.	284
chuck for stew, lean & fat, braised, 4 oz.	371
chuck for stew, lean, trimmed of fat, braised, 4 oz.	243
chuck, ground, lean, cooked, 4 oz.	315
chuck rib roast, lean, trimmed of fat, braised, 4 oz.	282
chuck roast, lean, trimmed of fat, cooked, 4 oz.	219
club steak, lean & fat, broiled, 4 oz.	517
club steak, lean, trimmed of fat, broiled, 4 oz.	278
flank steak (London broil), lean, trimmed of fat, pot roasted, 4 oz.	222
foreshank, lean, trimmed of fat, cooked, 4 oz.	210
ground, regular (21% fat), broiled, 4 oz.	324
ground, lean (10% fat), broiled, 4 oz.	248
porterhouse steak, lean & fat, broiled, 4 oz.	530
porterhouse steak, lean, trimmed of fat, broiled, 4 oz.	255
rib roast, lean & fat, roasted, 4 oz.	502
rib roast, lean, trimmed of fat, roasted 4 oz.	275

Food	*Calories*
round steak, lean & fat, broiled, 4 oz.	293
round steak, lean, trimmed of fat, broiled, 4 oz.	214
rump roast, lean & fat, roasted, 4 oz.	395
rump roast, lean, trimmed of fat, roasted, 4 oz.	236
sirloin steak, lean & fat, broiled, 4 oz.	465
sirloin steak, lean, trimmed of fat, broiled, 4 oz.	235
T-bone steak, lean & fat, broiled, 4 oz.	539
T-bone steak, lean, trimmed of fat, broiled, 4 oz.	253

Beef, corned

boiled, 4 oz.	424
canned, fatty, 4 oz.	301
canned, medium fat, 4 oz.	245
canned, lean, 4 oz.	211
hash, with potatoes, uncooked, 4 oz.	231

Beef, dried or chipped, creamed, ½ cup	210
Beef goulash, canned, 4 oz.	95

Beef suet

4 oz.	968
rendered, 1 tbsp.	120

Beef and vegetable stew, canned, 4 oz.	90

Beer (see beverages)

Beets

raw, peeled, diced, 1 cup	58
cooked, whole, peeled, 2 beets	32
canned, 1 cup, diced	63

Beet greens, cooked, 1 cup	26

Beverages (nonalcoholic)

cider, sweet, 8 oz.	125
cocoa, all milk, 1 cup	175

coffee

black, 1 cup	5
black with 1 tsp. sugar, 1 cup	35
with 1 tbsp. half & half, 1 cup	25
with 1 tbsp. light cream, 1 cup	35
with 1 tbsp. whole milk, 1 cup	15
with 1 tsp. sugar and 1 tbsp. cream	65

eggnog, all milk, 8 oz.	290
lemonade, 8 oz.	105

Food	*Calories*
milk	
buttermilk, 8 oz.	80
chocolate, 8 oz.	205
skim, 8 oz.	80
whole, 8 oz.	160
milk shake, chocolate, 8 oz.	420
milk shake, chocolate malted, 8 oz.	500
soft drinks	
cola, 12 oz.	144
cream soda, 12 oz.	156
fruit-flavored (orange, grape, etc.) 12 oz.	168
ginger ale, 12 oz.	109
root beer, 12 oz.	156
tea	
no sugar, 1 cup	0
with 1 tsp. lemon, 1 cup	5
with 1 tbsp. whole milk, 1 cup	10
with 1 tsp. sugar, 1 cup	30
Beverages (alcoholic)	
beer and ale	
ale, mild, 8 oz.	100
beer, regular, 12 oz.	156
beer, light, 12 oz.	104
distilled spirits	
brandy, 1 pony glass	70
cognac, 1 pony glass	70
gin, 86 proof, 1 jigger	105
gin, 100 proof, 1 jigger	124
rum, 80 proof, 1 jigger	97
rum, 100 proof, 1 jigger	124
vodka, 80 proof, 1 jigger	97
vodka, 100 proof, 1 jigger	124
whiskey, blended, 86 proof, 1 jigger	110
whiskey, bourbon, 86 proof, 1 jigger	110
whiskey, rye, 86 proof, 1 jigger	110
whiskey, Scotch, 86 proof, 1 jigger	110
liqueurs and cordials	
absinthe, 1 oz.	84

Food	Calories
anisette, 1 oz.	111
Benedictine, 1 oz.	112
brandy, fruit-flavored, 1 oz.	86
brandy, coffee, 1 oz.	88
brandy, ginger, 1 oz.	74
Cherry Heering, 1 oz.	80
crème de almond, 1 oz.	101
crème de banana, 1 oz.	96
crème de cacao, 1 oz.	101
crème de cassis, 1 oz.	83
crème de menthe, 1 oz.	110
Curaçao, 1 oz.	100
Drambuie, 1 oz.	110
kirsch, 1 oz.	83
kümmel, 1 oz.	75
maraschino, 1 oz.	94
peppermint schnapps, 1 oz.	83
Pernod, 1 oz.	79
sloe gin, 1 oz.	83
Southern Comfort, 1 oz.	120
triple sec, 1 oz.	83
vodka, fruit flavors, 1 oz.	100
mixed drinks	
daiquiri, 3.5 oz.	120
gin rickey, 1 glass	150
highball, 4 oz.	83
Manhattan, 3.5 oz.	165
martini, 3.5 oz.	140
old fashioned, 4 oz.	180
Tom Collins, 10 oz.	180
wines	
Beaujolais, 4 oz.	96
Bordeaux, 4 oz.	96
Burgundy, red, 4 oz.	96
Burgundy, sparkling, 4 oz.	116
Burgundy, white, 4 oz.	90
champagne, brut, 4 oz.	100
champagne, extra dry, 4 oz.	116

Food	Calories
Chianti, 4 oz.	100
Dubonnet, 4 oz.	160
liebfraumilch, 4 oz.	84
Madeira, 4 oz.	160
muscatel, 4 oz.	196
port, ruby, 4 oz.	184
Rhine, 4 oz.	96
Rhone, 4 oz.	96
Riesling, 4 oz.	90
rosé, 4 oz.	95
Sauternes, 4 oz.	110
sherry, 4 oz.	185
sherry, dry, 4 oz.	162
sherry, cream, 4 oz.	200
vermouth, French, 4 oz.	120
vermouth, Italian, 4 oz.	189

Biscuits
1 medium	130
1 small	85

Blackberries
fresh, 1 cup	85
canned, 1 cup with syrup	230
canned, water pack, 1 cup with liquid	100

Black-eyed peas (see cowpeas)

Blueberries
fresh, 1 cup	85
canned, water pack, 1 cup with liquid	90
canned, 1 cup with syrup	240
frozen, unsweetened, 1 cup	90

Bluefish
baked or broiled with butter, 4 oz.	180
fried, 4 oz.	232

Bologna (see sausage)

Bouillon, beef or chicken, 1 cube	5

Boysenberries
canned, water pack, 1 cup	88
frozen, unsweetened, 1 cup	60

Brains, all kinds, raw, 3 oz.	105

Food	*Calories*
Bran, added sugar, 1 cup	144
Branflakes, 1 cup	106
Braunschweiger (see sausage)	
Brazil nuts	
shelled, 1 cup	916
shelled, 1 oz. (8 medium)	185
Breads	
banana tea, 1 slice	135
Boston brown, 1 slice	95
bran raisin, 1 slice	150
corn, 1 piece (2 in.)	95
cracked wheat, 1 slice	66
French, 1 piece (2½ in.)	44
French, hoagie or submarine, 1 roll	392
Italian, 1 slice (4½ in.)	83
protein, 1 slice	45
pumpernickel, 1 slice	80
raisin, 1 slice	66
rye, American, light, 1 slice	55
rye, party sliced, 1 slice	40
salt rising, 1 slice	64
spoon, 1 serving	190
Vienna, 1 slice	73
white, 1 slice	74
whole wheat, 1 slice	56
Breads, fancy & sweet (½″ slice)	
banana-nut, 1 slice	71
chocolate-nut, 1 slice	87
date-nut, 1 slice	75
orange-nut, 1 slice	77
Breadcrumbs, 1 cup	392
Bread pudding, with raisins, 1 cup	496
Bread sticks, 5 sticks, large	192
Bread stuffing, 1 cup	416
Broad beans, mature seeds, dry, 2 oz.	192
Broccoli	
raw, 3 medium stalks (1 lb.)	145
cooked, 1 medium stalk	47

Food	*Calories*
cooked, stalks, ½ in. pieces, 1 cup	40
frozen, cooked, 1 cup	48
Brussels sprouts	
raw, 4 oz.	51
cooked, 1 cup	56
Buckwheat flour, light, sifted, 1 cup	340
Bulgur (parboiled wheat)	
dry, club wheat, 1 cup	628
canned, red winter wheat, 1 cup	227
Buns	
cinnamon, 1	160
cinnamon, raisin, 1	165
hot cross, 1	110
Butter	
regular, 1 cup	1,625
regular, 1 tbsp.	102
regular, 1 pat	36
whipped, 1 cup	1,081
whipped, 1 tbsp.	67
Buttermilk, 1 cup	88
Butternuts, shelled, 4 oz.	713

"C"

Cabbage	
regular, cooked, 1 cup	29
red, shredded, 1 cup	28
Chinese, cooked, 1 cup	8
Cakes (¹⁄₁₂ of cake or piece 3″ × 3″)	
angel food, 1 piece	161
Boston cream pie, 1 piece	311
caramel, iced, 1 piece	315
chocolate devil's food, iced, 1 piece	443
chocolate devil's food, iced, 1 cupcake	162
chocolate malt, iced, 1 piece	308
coconut, iced, 1 piece	220
coffee cake, iced, 1 piece	195
coffee cake, iced, with nuts, 1 piece	245

Food	*Calories*
cupcake, iced, 1	172
fruit cake, dark, 1 wedge	163
gingerbread, 1 piece	371
honey spice, iced, 1 piece	363
jelly roll, 1 slice	245
layer, 2 layers, white, iced, 1 piece	310
marble, iced, 1 piece	288
pound, 1 piece	142
sponge, 1 piece	196
white, iced, 1 piece	390
yellow, iced, 1 piece	365
Cake icings	
caramel, 1 cup	1,224
chocolate, 1 cup	1,034
chocolate fudge, 1 cup	1,172
coconut, 1 cup	604
white, 1 cup	1,199
Candied fruit (see individual listings)	
Candy	
brown-sugar fudge, 1 piece	105
butterscotch, 1 piece	20
candy corn, 10 pieces	51
caramel, 1 piece	43
chocolate	
bittersweet, 1 oz.	135
semisweet, 1 oz.	144
sweet, 1 oz.	150
milk, plain, 1 oz.	147
milk, with peanuts, 1 oz.	154
bar, 2 oz.	300
bar with nuts, 1 oz.	155
kisses, 1 oz.	150
mint, 3 small	120
fudge	
chocolate, 1 oz.	113
chocolate with nuts, 1 oz.	121
vanilla, 1 oz.	113
vanilla with nuts, 1 oz.	120

Food	Calories
gumdrops, 1 large or 8 small	35
hard, 1 piece	3
Hershey milk chocolate, 1½ oz.	210
Hershey milk chocolate, almond 1¾ oz.	210
jellybeans, 10	104
lollipop, 1 large	215
Mars bar, 1 oz.	160
Mars Milky Way, 1 oz.	120
Mars Three Musketeers, 1 oz.	120
marshmallows, 1 regular	23
marshmallow, chocolate, 1	45
Nestlés milk chocolate, 1 oz.	150
peanut bars, 1 oz.	146
peanut brittle	119
Cantaloupe	
½ melon	60
1 cup diced	70
Capicola, (see sausage)	
Carob flour, 1 cup	252
Carp, raw, 4 oz.	131
Carrots	
raw, 1	30
cooked, sliced, 1 cup	48
canned, 1 cup	69
Casaba melon (see muskmelon)	
Cashew nuts	
roasted in oil, 1 cup	785
9 medium	80
Catfish, 3½ oz.	105
Catsup (see ketchup)	
Cauliflower	
raw, buds, 1 cup	27
cooked, 1 cup	28
frozen, cooked, 1 cup	32
Caviar, sturgeon, granular, 1 tbsp.	42
Celery	
raw, 1 large stalk	7
raw, diced, 1 cup	20
cooked, diced, 1 cup	21

Food	*Calories*
Cereals	
All Bran, 1 cup	192
Alpha Bits, 1 cup	110
Apple Jacks, 1 cup	112
bran, ½ cup	95
bran flakes, 1 cup	130
bran flakes with raisin, 1 cup	145
Cap'n Crunch, 1 cup	151
Cheerios, 1⅛ cup	100
Cocoa Krispies, 1 cup	113
corn flakes, 1 cup	95
corn grits, cooked, 1 cup	120
Cream of Wheat, cooked, 1 cup	130
farina, cooked, 1 cup	140
Froot Loops, 1 cup	114
Grape nuts, ¼ cup	110
hominy, 1 cup	120
Kellogg's Special K, 1 cup	60
Kix, 1 cup	100
Life, 1 cup	142
Lucky Charms, 1 cup	97
Maypo, oat, cooked, ¾ cup	115
oatmeal, cooked, 1 cup	150
oatmeal, dry, 1 cup	310
Post Toasties, 1¼ cup	100
Product 19, 1 cup	110
puffed rice, 1 cup	50
Rice Krispies, 1 cup	105
rolled oats, cooked, 1 cup	150
shredded wheat, 1 oz.	85
Sugar Frosted Flakes, 1 cup	143
Sugar Pops, 1 cup	110
Sugar Smacks, 1 cup	110
Trix, 1 cup	112
Wheat Chex, ½ cup	100
Wheatena, cooked, ⅔ cup	100
Wheaties, 1 cup	105
Chard, Swiss, cooked, 1 cup	26

Food	Calories
Cheese	
American, processed 1 oz.	105
American with brick, processed, 1 oz.	101
American with muenster, processed, 1 oz.	100
blue, 1 oz.	104
brick, 1 oz.	105
brick, processed, 1 oz.	102
Camembert, domestic, 1 oz.	84
Cheddar, grated, 1 tbsp.	30
Cheddar, 1 oz.	111
Cheddar, shredded, 1 cup	450
cottage, creamed, ½ cup	120
cottage, creamed, 1 oz.	30
cottage, creamed, 1 tbsp.	17
cottage, uncreamed, ½ cup	98
cottage, uncreamed, 1 oz.	24
cottage, uncreamed, 1 tbsp.	14
cream, 1 oz.	106
Edam, 1 oz.	105
Gorgonzola, 1 oz.	112
Gouda, 1 oz.	108
Gruyère, 1 oz.	115
Liederkranz, 1 oz.	85
Limburger, 1 oz.	98
Monterey, 1 oz.	102
mozzarella, 1 oz.	79
muenster, 1 oz.	100
Neufchâtel, 1 oz.	71
nuworld, 1 oz.	104
old English, processed, 1 oz.	105
Parmesan, 1 oz.	110
Parmesan, grated, 1 tbsp.	29
pimento, American, processed, 1 oz.	104
Port-Salut, 1 oz.	100
provolone, 1 oz.	99
Romano, 1 oz.	110
Romano, grated 1 tbsp.	30
Roquefort, 1 oz.	110

Food	Calories
Swiss, domestic, 1 oz.	104
Swiss, processed, 1 oz.	95
Velveeta, 1 oz.	90
Cheese soufflé, 1 oz.	62
Cheese spread, American, 1 oz.	80
Cheese twists, 5 pieces	16
Cherimoya, 1 fruit	459
Cherries	
raw, sour red, 1 cup	90
raw, sweet, 10	47
candied, 10	119
canned, red sour, 1 cup	105
canned, red sweet, 1 cup	208
maraschino, 1	10
Chestnuts, shelled, 2 large	30
Chewing gum, 1 piece	5
Chicken	
broiled, 4 oz.	154
canned, boned, 4 oz.	225
fried, breast, 1	160
fried, drumstick, 1	88
fried, thigh, 1	122
fried, wing, 1	82
roasted, light meat, no skin, 4 oz.	207
roasted, dark meat, no skin, 4 oz.	209
Chicken à la King, 1 cup	468
Chicken fricassee, 1 cup	368
Chicken gizzards (see gizzards)	
Chicken pot pie, small pie	545
Chicken stew, canned, 4 oz.	93
Chickpeas, raw, 1 cup	720
Chicory, chopped, 1 cup	14
Chili con carne	
with beans, 1 cup	339
without beans, canned, 1 cup	512
Chili powder, 1 tbsp.	51
Chives, raw, 1 tbsp.	1
Chocolate (see candy)	

Food	Calories
Chocolate syrup	
light type, 1 tbsp.	23
fudge type, 1 tbsp.	62
Chop suey, 1 cup	300
Chow mein, chicken, 1 cup	255
Chutney, apple, 4 oz.	234
Cider (see beverages)	
Clams	
cherrystone, 6 large	56
littleneck, 5	56
steamers, 4 large, 9 small	80
canned, ½ cup with liquid	50
Clam dip, sour cream, 1 tsp.	8
Clam juice, 1 cup	20
Cocoa, (see beverages)	
Cocoa powder, 1 tbsp.	20
Coconut	
1 piece 2 × 2 × ½ in.	156
shredded, 1 cup	345
Codfish	
broiled, fillet, 4 oz.	192
canned, drained, 4 oz.	97
dried, salted, 4 oz.	148
Coffee (see beverages)	
Cola (see beverages)	
Cold cuts (see sausage)	
Coleslaw, 1 cup	155
Collards, cooked, 1 cup	59
Cookies	
Animal Crackers, 1	10
applesauce, 1	33
arrowroot, 1	20
black walnut, 1	25
brownies, with nuts, not iced, 1	97
butter, 1	23
butterscotch, icebox, 1	115
chocolate, 1	95
chocolate chip, 1	50

Food	Calories
chocolate fudge sandwich, 1	100
chocolate snap, 1	20
chocolate wafer, 1	13
coconut bar, 1	45
creme sandwich, 1	46
date and nut	75
fig bar	50
gingersnaps, 1	30
graham cracker, 1	30
graham cracker, chocolate covered, 1	60
lady fingers, 1	39
lemon snap, 1	17
macaroon, 1	90
marshmallow, chocolate coated, 1 medium	53
marshmallow, coconut coated, 1 large	74
molasses, 1	137
oatmeal, with raisins, 1	59
Oreo cream sandwich, 1	40
peanut butter, 1	55
raisin, 1	67
sandwich type, 1	75
shortbread, 1	37
sugar, 1	36
sugar wafers, 1	46
Swiss cream sandwich, 1	50
vanilla wafer, 1	19
Cooking oil (see oils)	
Corn	
cooked, 1 ear	70
cooked, 1 cup	137
canned, whole kernel, 1 cup	174
canned, creamed, 1 cup	210
frozen, cooked, 1 cup	130
Cornbread (see breads)	
Corn flour, 1 cup	431
Corn fritters, 1	132
Corn grits	
cooked, 1 cup	125
dry, 1 cup	579

Food	Calories
Cornmeal	
cooked, 1 cup	120
dry, 1 cup	530
Corn muffins (see muffins)	
Corn oil (see oil)	
Corn pudding, 1 cup	255
Cornstarch, 1 tbsp.	30
Corn syrup (see syrup)	
Cottage cheese (see cheese)	
Cottonseed oil, (see oils)	
Cowpeas, cooked, 1 cup	190
Crab	
canned, 4 oz.	116
cooked (steamed), 4 oz.	55
deviled, 4 oz.	213
fried, soft shell, 1	185
imperial, 4 oz.	167
Crabapple, 1 (3½ oz.)	70
Crackers	
animal, 1	12
butter, 1	15
cheese, 1 medium	15
graham, 1	30
graham, chocolate covered, 1	60
Holland rusk, 1	50
matzo, 1 6″ piece	80
Melba toast, 1	15
oyster, 10	30
Ritz, 1	15
rye wafer, 1	15
Ry-Krisp, 1	20
saltine, 1	15
soda, 1	30
Triscuit, 1	20
Wheat Thins, 1	10
Zwieback, 1 slice	30
Cranberries, raw, 1 cup	44
Cranberry juice, 6 oz.	124
Cranberry sauce, canned, 1 cup	404

Food	*Calories*
Cream	
half & half, 1 tbsp.	20
light, coffee, or table, ½ cup	253
light, coffee, or table, 1 tbsp.	32
light, whipping, 1 cup or 2 cups whipped	717
heavy, 1 cup or 2 cups whipped	838
sour, 1 cup	455
sour, 1 tbsp.	29
Cream puff, 1	303
Cress, garden, 1 cup cooked	50
Cress, water, 10 sprigs	5
Cucumber, 1 medium	15
Currants, 1 cup	65
Cusk, steamed, 1 oz.	30
Custard, baked, 1 cup	305
Custard, frozen (see ice cream)	

"D"

Dandelion greens, cooked, 1 cup	35
Dates	
pitted, 10	219
chopped, 1 cup	488
Deviled ham (see sausage)	
Dips	
bacon, 1 oz.	71
blue cheese, 1 oz.	69
clam, 1 oz.	67
onion, 1 oz.	70
Donuts	
cake, 1	125
jelly, 1	225
raised or yeast, 1	125
sugared or iced, 1	150
Duck, roasted, 1 slice	110

"E"

Éclairs, custard filling, chocolate icing, 1	239
Eel, smoked, 1 serving	165

Food	*Calories*
Eggs	
fresh, whole, 1 large	82
fresh, whites, 1	17
fresh, yolks, 1	59
boiled, 1 large	82
boiled, chopped, 1 cup	222
dried, 1 cup	640
dried, whites, 4 oz.	400
dried, yolks, 4 oz.	760
fried, 1 large	99
omelet (see scrambled)	
poached, 1 large	82
scrambled, 1 large	111
Eggnog (see beverages)	
Eggplant, cooked, 1 cup	38
Elderberries, fresh, ½ lb.	154
Endive, small pieces, 1 cup	10
Escarole	
7 small leaves	5
½ lb.	40

"F"

Farina (see cereals)	
Fennel, leaves, raw, ½ lb.	58
Figs, raw, 1 medium	40
Filberts (hazelnuts), shelled, 1 ounce (20 nuts)	180
Fish (see individual kinds)	
Fish cakes	
fried, 4 oz.	195
frozen, 4 oz.	306
Fish loaf, cooked, 4 oz.	141
Fish sticks, breaded, cooked, frozen, 1 stick	50
Flounder, baked with butter or margarine, 1 oz.	57
Flour	
enriched, 1 cup	450
cake, self-rising, 1 cup	380
corn, 1 cup sifted	405
rye, dark, 1 cup sifted	262

Food	Calories
rye, light, 1 cup sifted	286
wheat, all-purpose, 1 cup sifted	400
wheat, bread, 1 cup sifted	401
wheat, cake or pastry, 1 cup sifted	365
Frankfurters (see sausage)	
French toast, 1 slice	185
Frog legs, fried, 6 large	420
Frostings (see cake icings)	
Frozen custard (see ice cream)	
Fruit (see individual listings)	
Fruit cocktail	
water pack, 1 cup	91
syrup pack, 1 cup	194
Fruit salad	
canned, water pack, 1 cup	86
canned, syrup pack, 1 cup	191

"G"

Food	Calories
Garbanzos (see chickpeas)	
Garlic	
raw, 1 clove	4
raw, 1 ounce	28
Gelatin	
plain, 1 tablespoon	35
fruit flavors, prepared, ½ cup	80
fruit flavors, fruit added, 1 square	140
diet, ½ cup	8
Gin (see beverages)	
Ginger ale (see beverages)	
Gingerbread (see cakes)	
Ginger root	
fresh, 1 oz.	14
candied, 1 oz.	96
Gizzard, chicken, cooked, 4 oz.	168
Goose, roasted, 4 oz.	264
Gooseberries, raw, 1 cup	59
Granadilla (passion fruit), 1 fruit	16

Food	Calories
Grapefruit (pink, red, or white)	
fresh, ½ medium	40
fresh, sections with juice, 1 cup	94
canned, sections, water pack, 1 cup	73
canned, sections, syrup pack, 1 cup	178
Grapefruit juice (pink, red, or white)	
fresh, 1 cup	96
canned, unsweetened, 1 cup	101
canned, sweetened, 1 cup	133
frozen, unsweetened, 1 cup	101
frozen, sweetened, 1 cup	117
Grapefruit & orange juice blended	
canned, unsweetened, 1 cup	106
canned, sweetened, 1 cup	125
Grapefruit peel, candied, 1 oz.	90
Grapes	
American type, Concord, Delaware, etc. 10 grapes	18
American type, Concord, Delaware, etc. 1 cup	70
European type, Thompson, Emperor, etc. 10 grapes	34
European type, Thompson, Emperor, etc. 1 cup	107
canned, water pack, 1 cup	125
canned, syrup pack, 1 cup	197
Grape drink, (30% juice), 1 cup	135
Grape juice	
canned or bottled, 1 cup	167
frozen concentrate, 1 cup	133
Gravy	
beef, canned, ½ cup	60
chicken, canned, ½ cup	108
chicken giblet, canned, ½ cup	56
mushroom, canned, ½ cup	60
brown, from mix, ½ cup	36
chicken, from mix, ½ cup	52
mushroom, from mix, ½ cup	48
onion, frozen mix, ½ cup	36
Griddle cakes (see pancakes)	
Grits, (see corn grits)	
Ground cherries (cape gooseberries), raw, 1 cup	74

Food	Calories
Grouper, raw, 4 oz.	99
Guavas, fresh, 1 small	48
Guinea hen, cooked, 4 oz.	177
Gum (see chewing gum)	

"H"

Haddock	
fried, 4 oz.	188
smoked, 4 oz.	117
Halibut	
broiled with butter or margarine, 4 oz.	192
smoked, 4 oz.	254
Ham (see pork)	
Hamburger, (see beef, ground)	
Hash, corned beef (see beef, corned)	
Hazelnuts (see filberts)	
Headcheese, (see sausage)	
Heart (cooked)	
beef, 1 oz.	53
calf, 1 oz.	59
chicken, 1 oz.	49
hog, 1 oz.	55
lamb, 1 oz.	74
turkey, 1 oz.	61
Herbs	0
Herring	
canned, 1 oz.	59
canned, in tomato sauce, 1 oz.	50
pickled, Bismarck, 1 herring	112
pickled, 1 oz.	63
smoked, kippered, canned, 1 medium fillet	84
smoked, kippered, canned, 1 oz.	60
Hickory nuts, shelled, 4 oz.	767
Hollandaise sauce, ½ cup	59
Hominy grits (see corn grits)	
Honey	
strained or extracted, 1 tbsp.	64
strained or extracted, 1 oz.	86

Food	Calories
Honeydew melon (see muskmelon)	
Horseradish	
raw, 1 oz.	18
prepared, 1 tbsp.	6
Huckleberries, 1 cup	85
Hyacinth beans, seeds, dry, 4 oz.	383

"I"

Ice	
orange, ¼ pint	70
twin pop bar	95
Ice Cream	
chocolate, ⅓ pint	191
strawberry, ⅓ pint	174
vanilla, ⅓ pint	180
vanilla fudge, ⅓ pint	183
French, chocolate, ⅓ pint	250
French, vanilla, ⅓ pint	247
frozen custard, plain, 1 cup	334
sherbet, orange, ⅓ pint	152
Ice cream bar, chocolate covered, 3 oz. bar	150
Ice cream cone	
sugar, 1 cone	37
waffle, 1 cone	19
Ice cream parfait, coffee, 1	260
Ice cream sandwich, 1	208
Ice cream soda, chocolate, vanilla ice cream, 8 oz.	255
Ice milk, vanilla, ⅓ pint	135
Ice milk bar, chocolate covered	144
Icings (see cake icings)	

"J"

Jackfruit, fresh, 4 oz.	31
Jams	
assorted, 1 tbsp.	54
assorted, 1 oz.	77
Jellies	
assorted, 1 tbsp.	55
assorted, 1 oz.	78

Food	Calories
Juice (see individual listings)	
Jujube, fresh, 4 oz.	111
Junket, with whole milk, ½ cup	115

"K"

Kale	
raw, 4 oz.	80
cooked, 1 cup	43
Ketchup	
1 tbsp.	20
1 oz.	30
Kidney, beef, cooked	286
Kingfish, raw, 4 oz.	119
Knockwurst (see sausage)	
Kohlrabi	
raw, diced, 1 cup	41
boiled, 1 cup	40
Kumquats, 1 medium	12

"L"

Lamb	
leg, roasted, lean, trimmed of fat, 4 oz.	211
leg, roasted, lean & fat, 4 oz.	317
loin chops, lean, trimmed of fat, 4 oz.	213
loin chops, lean & fat, 4 oz.	407
rib chops, lean, trimmed of fat, 4 oz.	239
rib chops, lean & fat, 4 oz.	462
shoulder, lean, trimmed of fat, 4 oz.	233
shoulder, lean & fat, 4 oz.	383
Lard	
1 lb.	4,091
1 cup	1,849
1 tbsp.	117
Leeks, raw, 1 average	17
Lemon, peeled, 1 medium	20
Lemonade, frozen concentrate, diluted with water, 6 oz.	81

Food	Calories
Lemon juice	
fresh, 1 cup	61
fresh, 1 tbsp.	4
canned, unsweetened, 1 cup	56
canned, unsweetened, 1 tbsp.	3
frozen, unsweetened, 1 tbsp.	3
Lemon peel	
raw, grated, 1 tbsp.	0
candied, 1 oz.	90
Lentils	
whole, raw, 1 cup	646
whole, cooked, 1 cup	212
split, raw, 1 cup	656
Lettuce (fresh)	
Boston or bibb, 1 head	23
Boston or bibb, 1 large leaf	2
iceberg (New York, Great Lakes), 1 head	70
iceberg (New York, Great Lakes), 3 leaves	6
iceberg (New York, Great Lakes), ½ lb.	28
romaine (white Paris), ½ lb.	41
romaine (white Paris), chopped, 1 cup	10
Simpson or looseleaf, ½ lb.	41
Simpson or looseleaf, chopped, 1 cup	10
Lima beans (see beans, lima)	
Limes, fresh, 1 lime	19
Limeade, frozen concentrate, diluted with water, 1 cup	102
Lime juice	
fresh, 1 cup	64
fresh, 1 tbsp.	4
canned, unsweetened, 1 cup	64
canned, unsweetened, 1 tbsp.	4
Litchi nuts	
raw, ¼ lb.	44
dried, 6 nuts	41
Liver (cooked)	
beef, 4 oz.	260
calf, 4 oz.	296

Food	Calories
chicken, 4 oz.	187
hog, 4 oz.	273
lamb, 4 oz.	296
turkey, 4 oz.	197
Liver paste, (pâté de foie gras), canned, 1 tbsp.	60
Liverwurst, (see sausage)	
Lobster	
northern, cooked, 1 cup	138
northern, cooked, 1 lb.	431
Lobster Newburg, 1 cup	485
Lobster paste, 1 oz.	51
Lobster salad, with tomatoes, 5 oz.	275
Loganberries, fresh, 1 cup	89
Loquats, fresh, 10 fruits	59
Lox, 4 oz.	200
Luncheon meats (see sausage)	

"M"

Food	Calories
Macadamia nuts, shelled, 6 nuts	106
Macaroni (enriched or unenriched)	
dry, 4 oz.	419
cooked, yield from 4 oz. dry (2⅕ cups)	419
cooked, 4 oz.	126
cooked, 1 cup	155
Macaroni & cheese	
baked, 1 cup	430
baked, 4 oz.	244
canned, 1 cup	228
canned, 4 oz.	108
Mackerel	
Atlantic, broiled with butter or margarine, 1 fillet	248
Atlantic, broiled with butter or margarine, 4 oz.	268
Pacific, canned, 4 oz.	204
salted, 1 fillet	342
salted, 4 oz.	344
Malt, dry, 1 oz.	104
Malt extract, dried, 1 oz.	104
Mamey (mammee apple), 1 fruit	446

Food	Calories
Mandarin oranges (see tangerines)	
Mangoes	
fresh, whole, 1 fruit	152
fresh, sliced, 1 cup	109
fresh, 4 oz.	75
Margarine	
regular, 1 stick, 4 oz.	816
regular, 1 pat	36
regular or soft, 1 cup	1,634
regular or soft, 1 tbsp.	102
Marmalade	
citrus, 1 tbsp.	51
citrus, 1 oz.	73
Marshmallow (see candy)	
Matai (see water chestnut, Chinese)	
Mayonnaise (see salad dressings)	
Meatloaf (see sausage)	
Meats (see beef, lamb, pork, veal)	
Melba toast, 1 slice	25
Melons (see muskmelons & watermelon)	
Milk, cow	
whole (3.5% fat), 1 cup	159
whole (3.5% fat), 4 oz.	80
skim, 1 cup	88
skim, 4 oz.	44
low fat (2% fat), 1 cup	145
low fat (2% fat), 4 oz.	73
canned, evaporated, 1 oz.	43
canned, condensed, 1 oz.	123
dry, regular, 1 cup	643
dry, instant, 1 cup	351
dry, nonfat, regular, 1 cup	436
dry, nonfat, instant, with water, 1 cup	80
malted, dry powder, 1 oz.	116
chocolate (see beverages)	
Milk, goat, 1 cup	163
Milk, human, 1 oz.	24
Milk, reindeer, 1 cup	580

Food	Calories
Milk shake (see beverages)	
Mint, chopped, 1 tbsp.	0
Mixed vegetables (see vegetables, mixed)	
Molasses, cane	
light, 1 tbsp.	50
light, 1 oz.	103
medium, 1 tbsp.	46
medium, 1 oz.	95
blackstrap, 1 tbsp.	43
blackstrap, 1 oz.	87
Barbados, 1 tbsp.	54
Barbados, 1 oz.	111
Mortadella (see sausage)	
Muffins (enriched or unenriched flour)	
plain, 1 muffin	118
blueberry, 1 muffin	112
bran, 1 muffin	104
corn, 1 muffin	126
Mushrooms	
sliced, 1 cup	20
1 oz.	8
Muskmelons	
cantaloupe, ½ melon	82
cantaloupe, cubed or melon balls, 1 cup	48
cantaloupe, 4 oz.	34
casaba (Golden Beauty), ½ melon	184
casaba (Golden beauty), cubed or melon balls, 1 cup	46
casaba (Golden Beauty), 4 oz.	31
honeydew, ½ melon	248
honeydew, cubed or melon balls, 1 cup	56
honeydew, 4 oz.	38
frozen melon balls in syrup, 1 cup	143
Mussels, raw, 4 oz. of meat only	108
Mustard (prepared)	
brown, 1 tsp.	5
brown, 1 cup	228

Food	Calories
yellow, 1 tsp.	4
yellow, 1 cup	188
Mustard greens	
raw, 4 oz.	35
cooked (boiled), 1 cup	32
frozen, cooked, 1 cup	30
Mustard spinach (tendergreen)	
raw, 4 oz.	25
cooked, 1 cup	29
Mutton (see lamb)	

"N"

Nectarines, fresh, 1 medium	88
Noodles (enriched or unenriched)	
egg, dry, 4 oz.	440
egg, cooked, 1 cup	200
chow mein, canned, 3 oz.	416
chow mein, canned, 1 cup	220
Nuts (see individual kinds)	
Nuts, mixed, 8–12	95

"O"

Oats	
oat flakes, maple flavored, cooked, 1 cup	166
oat granules, maple flavored, cooked, 1 cup	147
oat & wheat cereal, cooked, 1 cup	159
oatmeal (see cereal)	
shredded oats, 1 cup	171
puffed oats, 1 cup	99
Ocean perch (Atlantic)	
fried, 4 oz.	256
frozen, breaded, fried, 1 fillet	281
frozen, breaded, fried, 4 oz.	362
Oils	
corn, safflower, soybean, cottonseed, 1 cup	1,927
corn, safflower, soybean, cottonseed, 1 tbsp.	120
olive, peanut, 1 cup	1,909
olive, peanut, 1 tbsp.	119

Food	*Calories*
Okra	
raw, sliced, 1 cup	36
cooked, sliced, 1 cup	46
frozen, cooked, sliced, 1 cup	70
Oleomargarine (see margarine)	
Olives	
green, 5 small	16
ripe, Ascolane, 5 large	30
ripe, Manzanillo, 5 small	19
ripe, Mission, 5 small	27
ripe, Sevillano, 5 large	32
Olive oil (see oils)	
Omelet (see eggs, omelet)	
Onions	
fresh, chopped, 1 cup	65
fresh, minced, 1 tbsp.	4
cooked (boiled), sliced, 1 cup	61
whole, 1 average	40
Onion rings, frozen, 4 oz.	146
Oranges	
navels, 1 medium	71
Valencia, 1 medium	62
Florida, 1 medium	71
sections, 1 cup	88
diced, small pieces, 1 cup	103
Orange juice	
fresh, navel, 1 cup	120
fresh, Valencia, 1 cup	117
fresh, Florida, 1 cup	106
fresh, all varieties, juice from 1 orange	39
canned, unsweetened, 1 cup	120
canned, sweetened, 1 cup	130
frozen, concentrate, mixed with water, 1 cup	122
Orange juice drink, commercial, powder with water, 8 oz.	118
Orange peel	
raw, grated, 1 tbsp.	0
candied, 1 oz.	90

Food	Calories
Orange-apricot juice drink (40% juices), 1 cup	125
Orange-pineapple drink, commercial, 8 oz.	117
Oyster plant (see Salsify)	
Oysters	
raw, Easter, 1 cup (13–19 medium)	158
raw, Pacific and Olympia, 1 cup (4–6 medium)	218
cooked (fried), 4 medium	108
scalloped, 6	355
Oyster stew, 1 part oyster, 2 parts milk, 1 cup	233

"P"

Food	Calories
Pancakes	
plain & buttermilk, 1 small (2 tbsp. batter)	61
plain & buttermilk, 1 large (7 tbsp. batter)	164
buckwheat, 1 small (2 tbsp. batter)	54
buckwheat, 1 large (7 tbsp. batter)	146
Papaws, whole, 1	83
Papaya	
1 medium (1 lb.)	119
cubed, ½ cup	36
Parfait, (see ice cream, parfait)	
Parsley	
chopped, 1 tbsp.	2
10 sprigs	4
Parsnips	
raw, ½ lb.	146
cooked, diced, 1 cup	102
Passion fruit (see granadilla)	
Pastina, egg, dry, 1 cup	651
Pastries	
cream puff, 1	295
Danish, 1 small	150
éclair, chocolate custard	315
Pastry shell (see pie crust)	
Pâté de fois gras, 1 tbsp.	60
Peaches	
fresh, whole, 1 medium	38
fresh, sliced, 1 cup	70

Food	*Calories*
canned, water pack, 1 cup	76
canned, syrup pack, 1 cup	200
dehydrated, cooked with sugar, 1 cup	351
dried, sulfured, uncooked, 1 cup	419
frozen, sliced, 1 cup	220
Peach nectar, canned, 1 cup	120
Peanuts	
roasted in shell, shelled, 10 nuts	105
roasted, shelled, chopped, 1 tbsp.	52
roasted, shelled, chopped, 1 cup	838
roasted, shelled, 1 oz.	166
Peanut butter	
1 cup	1,520
1 tbsp.	94
Peanut flour, defatted	223
Peanut oil (see oils)	
Pears	
fresh, Bartlett, 1 medium	100
fresh, Bosc, 1 medium	86
fresh, sliced, 1 cup	101
canned, water pack, 1 cup	78
canned, syrup pack, 1 cup	194
candied, 1 oz.	86
dried, sulfured, uncooked, 1 cup	482
Pear nectar, canned, 1 cup	130
Peas, black-eyed (see cowpeas)	
Peas, green	
boiled, drained, ½ cup	57
canned, ½ cup with liquid	82
canned, drained, ½ cup	70
frozen, ½ cup	69
frozen, with butter sauce, ½ cup	99
frozen, with cream sauce. ½ cup	89
Peas, split, boiled, drained, ½ cup	115
Peas and carrots, frozen, cooked, ½ cup	43
Pecans	
shelled, 10 medium	96
shelled, 1 cup	742

Food	Calories
chopped, 1 tbsp.	52
chopped, 1 cup	811
Peppers, hot, chili	
canned in chili sauce, 1 cup	51
dried, 1 tsp.	7
Peppers, sweet	
green, fresh, sliced, 1 cup	18
green, boiled, sliced, 1 cup	24
red, fresh, sliced, 1 cup	25
red, whole, fresh, 1 medium	19
Perch (see ocean perch)	
Persimmons	
Japanese, 1	129
North American, 1	31
Pickles	
dill, whole, 1 medium	7
dill, sliced, 1 cup	17
fresh, sweetened, sliced, 1 cup	124
sour, whole, 1 medium	7
sweet, Gherkins, whole, 1 small	22
sweet, chopped, ½ cup	117
chow-chow, sour, 1 cup	70
chow-chow, sweet, 1 cup	284
relish, sweet, 1 tbsp.	21
relish, sweet, 1 cup	338
Pies (baked, 4¾ in. arc)	
apple	404
banana cream	350
banana custard	336
blackberry	384
blueberry	382
Boston cream (see cakes)	
butterscotch	406
cherry	412
chocolate chiffon	354
chocolate meringue	383
coconut custard	357
custard	331

Food	Calories
lemon chiffon	338
lemon meringue	357
mince	428
peach	403
pecan	577
pineapple	400
pineapple chiffon	311
pineapple custard	334
pumpkin	321
raisin	427
rhubarb	400
shoo-fly	440
strawberry	246
strawberry cream	380
sweet potato	324
Pies, frozen (⅙ pie)	
apple	255
cherry	259
chocolate cream	289
Pie crust, baked, 1 pie shell	900
Pignolias (see pine nuts)	
Pigs' feet, pickled, 2 oz.	113
Pike, raw	
blue, 4 oz.	102
northern, 4 oz.	100
wall-eye, 4 oz.	106
Pilinuts, shelled, ½ lb.	1,518
Pimientos	
canned, 4 oz.	31
1 medium	10
Pineapple	
fresh, diced, 1 cup	81
fresh, sliced, 1 slice	44
candied, 1 oz.	90
canned, water pack, 1 cup	96
canned, heavy syrup, 1 cup	189
canned, extra heavy syrup, 1 cup	234
frozen, sweetened, chunks, 1 cup	208

Food	*Calories*
Pineapple juice	
canned, unsweetened, 1 cup	138
frozen, concentrate, with water, 1 cup	130
Pineapple juice and grapefruit juice, drink	
(50% juices) 1 cup	135
Pineapple juice and orange juice, drink	
(40% juices) 1 cup	135
Pine nuts, pignolias, shelled, 1 oz.	156
Pine nuts, piñon, shelled, 1 oz.	180
Pistachio nuts	
shelled, ¼ lb.	674
shelled, ½ cup	446
chopped, 1 tbsp.	53
Pitanga (Surinam cherry), 2 fruits	5
Pizza	
baked, cheese, ⅛ of 14-in. diam. pie	153
baked, sausage & cheese, ⅛ of 14-in. diam. pie	157
frozen, baked, commercial, cheese,	
⅐ of 10-in. diam. pie	139
Plantain (baking banana), raw, 1 medium	313
Plums	
fresh, damson, 1 cup	87
fresh, damson, 1 medium (2″ diam.)	36
Japanese, 1 medium (2⅛″ diam.)	32
prune type, 1 medium (1½″ diam.)	21
canned, purple, water pack, 1 cup	114
canned, purple, syrup pack, 1 cup	214
Pokeberry shoots, cooked, 1 cup	33
Pomegranate, 1 medium	97
Pompano, medium piece	170
Popcorn	
unpopped, 1 cup	742
popped, plain, 1 cup	23
popped in oil, 1 cup	41
popped in oil, with 1 tbsp. butter or margarine,	
1 cup	143
popped, sugar coated, 1 cup	134
Popovers, 1 medium	60

Food	Calories
Porgy, 4 oz.	126
Pork (fresh or cured)	
bacon (see bacon)	
ham, boiled, 4 oz.	266
ham, fresh, medium-fat, roasted, 4 oz.	426
ham, light-cure, medium-fat, roasted, 4 oz.	329
ham, light-cure, lean only, roasted, 4 oz.	213
ham, long-cure, country style, medium-fat, 4 oz.	443
ham, long-cure, country style, lean only, 4 oz.	353
ham, minced, 4 oz.	259
ham, picnic, cured, medium-fat, roasted, 4 oz.	368
ham, picnic, cured, lean only, roasted, 4 oz.	241
ham, canned, deviled, 4 oz.	398
ham, canned, spiced, 4 oz.	336
loin roast, lean & fat, baked, 4 oz.	411
loin roast, lean, trimmed of fat, baked, 4 oz.	288
loin chops, lean & fat, broiled, 4 oz.	454
loin chops, lean, trimmed of fat, broiled, 4 oz.	302
Boston butt, lean & fat, roasted, 4 oz.	400
Boston butt, lean, trimmed of fat, roasted, 4 oz.	277
picnic, lean & fat, cooked, 4 oz.	424
picnic, lean, trimmed of fat, cooked, 4 oz.	241
spareribs, lean meat with fat, braised, 4 oz.	500
Pork sausage (see sausage)	
Pork and beans, ½ cup	160
Potatoes	
fresh, peeled, 1 medium	86
fresh, peeled, chopped, 1 cup	114
fresh, peeled, ½ lb.	173
baked, 1 medium	145
baked, ½ lb.	163
boiled, 1 medium	104
boiled, ½ lb.	173
French fried, 10 strips	200
French fried, 4 oz.	311
fried, 1 cup	456
hashed brown, 1 cup	355
mashed, with milk, 1 cup	137

Food	Calories
scalloped & au gratin, with cheese, 1 cup	355
scalloped & au gratin, without cheese, 1 cup	255
dehydrated mashed, flakes with milk & table fat, 1 cup	195
frozen (diced, shredded, or crinkle cut) cooked, 1 cup	347
frozen, French fried, 17 pieces	187
sweet potatoes (see sweet potatoes)	
Potato chips	
10 chips	114
1 oz.	161
Potato salad	
regular, 1 cup	248
regular, with mayonnaise & French dressing, 1 cup	363
Potato sticks, 1 oz.	154
Pretzels	
Dutch, 1 large	60
10 sticks or 1 three-ring	10
Prickly pear, raw, 4 oz.	46
Prunes	
dehydrated, uncooked, 1 cup	344
dehydrated, cooked, with sugar, 1 cup	504
dried, uncooked, 4 oz.	250
dried, uncooked, 1 medium	19
dried, cooked, without sugar, 1 cup	253
Prune juice, bottled, or canned, 1 cup (8 oz.)	197
Prune whip, baked, hot, 1 cup	140
Puddings, prepared commercial brands	
banana, ½ cup	165
Bavarian cream, orange, ½ cup	290
blanc mange, ½ cup	140
bread, ½ cup	210
butterscotch, ½ cup	190
chocolate, ½ cup	190
custard, ½ cup	145
Indian, ½ cup	121
lemon, ½ cup	125
lemon chiffon, ½ cup	144

Food	*Calories*
rice, ½ cup	140
tapioca, chocolate, ½ cup	185
tapioca, vanilla, ½ cup	170
vanilla, ½ cup	165
Puddings, instant commercial brands	
banana cream, ½ cup	175
butterscotch, ½ cup	175
caramel, ½ cup	195
chocolate, ½ cup	185
lemon, ½ cup	180
mocha, ½ cup	200
vanilla, ½ cup	180
Pumpkin	
fresh, ½ lb.	42
canned, 1 cup	81
Pumpkin seeds (& squash seeds), dry, hulled,	
½ cup	387

"Q"

Quail, fresh, 4 oz.	172
Quinces, fresh, 4 oz.	79

"R"

Rabbit, stewed, 4 oz.	245
Radishes	
fresh, 10 medium	8
fresh, sliced, ½ cup	5
Raisins	
fresh, packaged, 1 tbsp.	26
fresh, packaged, 1 cup (not packed)	419
cooked, with sugar, 1 cup	628
Raspberries	
red, fresh, 1 pint	185
red, fresh, 1 cup	70
red, frozen, sweetened, 1 cup	245
red, canned, water pack, 1 cup	85
black, fresh, 1 cup	98
Redfish (see ocean perch)	
Relish (see pickles)	

Food	Calories
Rennin	
tablet, 1	12
dessert from tablet, 1 cup	227
chocolate dessert from milk, 1 cup	260
desserts from milk (caramel, vanilla, etc.), 1 cup	238
Rhubarb	
fresh, diced, 1 cup	20
cooked, with sugar, 1 cup	381
frozen, sweetened, 1 cup	386
Rice (enriched or unenriched)	
brown, long grain, raw, 1 cup	666
brown, long grain, cooked, 1 cup	232
white, long grain, milled, raw, 1 cup	672
white, long grain, milled, cooked, 1 cup	223
white, medium grain, milled, raw, 1 cup	708
white, long grain, instant, cooked, 1 cup	180
spanish, cooked, 1 cup	130
Rice mixes (commercial)	
beef, 1 cup	320
chicken, 1 cup	314
wild, 1 cup	282
Rice pudding, with raisins, 1 cup	387
Rockfish	
steamed, 1 fillet	123
steamed, 4 oz.	120
Roe, herring, canned, 4 oz.	134
Rolls and buns	
brown & serve, baked, 1	84
cloverleaf roll, 1	119
Danish pastry, plain, 1	317
hard roll, Kaiser, 1	156
hoagie or submarine roll, 1 large	392
frankfurter roll, 1	119
hamburger bun, 1	119
sweet roll, 1	180
whole wheat roll, 1	90
Romaine (see lettuce)	
Root beer (see beverages)	

Food	*Calories*
Rum (see beverages)	
Rusk, 1	38
Rutabagas	
raw, cubed, 1 cup	64
cooked, cubed, 1 cup	60
Rye flour, light, sifted, 1 cup	314
Rye wafers, 1	23

"S"

Safflower oil (see oil)	
Salad dressings	
blue cheese, 1 tbsp.	76
blue cheese, dietary, 1 tbsp.	12
French, 1 tbsp.	66
French, dietary, 1 tbsp.	15
Italian, 1 tbsp.	83
Italian, dietary, 1 tbsp.	8
mayonnaise, 1 tbsp.	101
Roquefort, 1 tbsp.	76
Roquefort, dietary, 1 tbsp.	12
Russian, 1 tbsp.	74
salad dressing, mayonnaise type, 1 tbsp.	65
salad dressing, mayonnaise type, dietary, 1 tbsp.	22
Thousand Island, 1 tbsp.	80
Thousand Island, dietary, 1 tbsp.	27
vinegar and oil, equal parts, 1 tbsp.	65
Salad oil (see oils)	
Salads	
apple-carrot, ½ cup	100
apple, celery, & walnut (½ cup)	135
avocado, ½ cup	130
carrot-raisin, 3 tbsp.	155
coleslaw (see coleslaw)	
chicken with celery, 3 tbsp.	180
combination vegetable, 1 cup	75
crab with celery, 3 tbsp.	135
egg and tomato (½ of each)	65
endive with dressing, ½ cup	230

Food	*Calories*
fruit, mixed, canned, 3 tbsp.	150
gelatin (see gelatin)	
lettuce and tomatoes, 4 leaves & 1 small tomato	35
lobster, ½ cup	110
macaroni, ½ cup	167
potato (see potato salad)	
tomato and cucumber, 1 of each	40
tuna, 1 serving	170
Salami (see sausage)	
Salmon	
Atlantic, canned, 4 oz.	230
chinook (king), canned, 4 oz.	238
chum, canned, 4 oz.	158
coho (silver), canned, 4 oz.	174
pink (humpback), canned, 4 oz.	160
sockeye (red), canned, 4 oz.	194
broiled with butter or margarine, 4 oz.	208
smoked, 4 oz.	200
Salmon rice loaf, 4 oz.	138
Salsify, cooked, cubed, 1 cup	50
Salt	0
Sandwiches (on white bread, plain, 1 sandwich)	
anchovy/cream cheese (5 fillets, 1 oz. cheese)	232
anchovy/pimiento (5 fillets, 3 pimientos)	157
bacon (4 slices)	288
bacon/cheese (4 slices bacon, 1 oz. American cheese)	399
bacon/egg (4 slices bacon, ½ hard-cooked egg)	329
bacon, lettuce, tomato (4 slices bacon)	280
bologna (2 oz.)	248
bologna/cheese (2 oz. bologna, 1 oz. cheese)	355
cheese, American or Cheddar (2 oz.)	314
cheese, cream/jelly (2 oz. cheese, 1 tbsp. jelly)	357
cheese, Swiss (2 oz.)	300
chicken, 2 oz. roasted meat	196
chicken salad, 2 oz.	245
club (bacon, chicken, tomato, lettuce, 3 slices bread)	590

Food	Calories
corned beef (2 oz. boiled meat)	304
cucumber/tomato (½ of each)	124
egg, fried (1 egg)	206
egg salad	280
egg/tomato (½ hard cooked egg, ½ tomato)	150
ham, boiled (2 oz.)	225
ham/cheese (2 oz. boiled ham, 1 oz. cheese)	336
ham, deviled (2 oz.)	291
ham, minced (2 oz.)	222
ham salad	320
hamburger (2 oz. broiled meat)	255
hamburger/cheese (2 oz. meat, 1 oz. cheese)	366
herring, tomato (2 oz.)	192
jelly (2 tbsp.)	202
lettuce/tomato (3 leaves, ½ tomato)	115
liverwurst	267
liverwurst/cheese (2 oz. meat, 1 oz. cheese)	375
peanut butter (2 tbsp.)	292
peanut butter/cream cheese (2 tbsp. peanut buter, 1 tbsp. cheese)	348
peanut butter/jelly (2 tbsp. peanut butter, 1 tbsp. jelly)	347
roast beef (2 oz. meat)	241
salami (2 oz.)	269
salami/cheese (2 oz. salami, 1 oz. cheese)	380
salami/egg (2 oz. salami, 1 fried egg)	383
salmon, smoked (2 oz.)	192
salmon, smoked with 1 oz. cream cheese	297
sardines (2 oz.)	187
sardines/cream cheese (2 oz. sardines, 1 oz. cheese)	292
tongue, beef (2 oz.)	231
tuna salad	280
turkey (2 oz. roasted meat)	200
watercress/cream cheese (10 sprigs cress, 1 oz. cheese)	199
Sandwich spread, 1 tbsp.	57
Sandwich spread, dietary, 1 tbsp.	17

Food	*Calories*
Sardines	
Atlantic, canned in oil, with liquid, 4 oz.	352
Atlantic, canned in oil, drained, 4 oz.	232
Atlantic, canned in oil, drained, 1 medium fish	24
Pacific, canned in brine or mustard, 4 oz.	224
Pacific, canned in tomato sauce, 4 oz.	224
Sauces	
barbecue, 1 tbsp.	17
butterscotch, 1 tbsp.	100
cheese, ¼ cup	130
chili, 1 tbsp.	15
chocolate, 1 tbsp.	45
cream, 1 tbsp.	35
custard, ¼ cup	85
fudge, 1 tbsp.	50
garlic, with butter, 1 tbsp.	100
Hollandaise, ¼ cup	185
hot pepper, 1 tbsp.	3
lemon, ¼ cup	135
raisin, ¼ cup	125
sour cream, ¼ cup	140
soy, 1 cup	197
soy, 1 tbsp.	10
tartar, 1 tbsp.	95
tomato, canned, ¼ cup	30
white, medium, ¼ cup	110
Worcestershire, 1 tbsp.	10
Sauerkraut, canned, 1 cup	42
Sauerkraut juice, canned, 1 cup	24
Sausage, cold cuts, luncheon meats	
blood sausage, 1 oz.	112
bockwurst, 1 link	172
bockwurst, 1 oz.	75
bologna, chub, ⅛″ slice	40
bologna, ring, 1⅜″ ring	1,034
bologna, slices, 1 slice, 1 oz.	86
Braunschweiger (liverwurst), 1 oz.	90
Braunschweiger (liverwurst), 1 slice (¼″ thick)	90

Food	Calories
brown & serve sausage, cooked, 1 patty	97
brown & serve sausage, cooked, 1 link	72
brown & serve sausage, cooked, 1 oz.	120
capicola, packaged, 1 slice	105
capicola, packaged, 1 oz.	141
cervelat, packaged, 1 oz.	128
country-style sausage, 1 oz.	98
deviled ham, canned, 1 tbsp.	46
deviled ham, canned, 1 oz.	100
frankfurters, chilled, 1 (2 oz.)	176
frankfurters, smoked, chilled, 1 (1.5 oz.)	124
frankfurters, cooked, 1 (2 oz.)	170
frankfurters, cooked, 1 oz.	85
headcheese, 1 slice (1 oz.)	76
knockwurst, 4″ link, 1 link	189
knockwurst, 1 oz.	79
liverwurst (see sausage, Braunschweiger)	
luncheon meat, boiled ham, 1 oz.	66
luncheon meat, chopped pork, 1 oz.	83
meatloaf, 1 oz.	57
minced ham, 1 oz.	65
mortadella, 1 slice	79
mortadella, 1 oz.	89
Polish sausage, 1 sausage (1″ diam., 5.5″ long)	240
Polish sausage, 1 oz.	86
pork sausage, cooked, 1 link	62
pork sausage, cooked, 1 oz.	134
pork sausage, canned, drained, 1 oz.	108
salami, dry, 1 oz.	128
salami, cooked, 1 oz.	88
scrapple, 1 oz.	61
Thuringer cervelat (summer sausage), 1 oz.	87
Vienna, canned, 1 oz.	68
Scallions (see onions)	
Scallops (bay & sea)	
cooked (steamed), 4 oz.	127
frozen, breaded, cooked, 4 oz.	220
Scrapple (see sausage)	

Food	Calories
Sesame seeds	
dry, hulled, 1 tbsp.	47
dry, hulled, 1 cup	873
Shad, baked, 4 oz.	228
Shallot bulbs, raw, chopped, 1 tbsp.	7
Sherbet (see ice cream)	
Shortbread (see cookies)	
Shortcake, strawberry, medium serving	400
Shortening, 1 tbsp.	100
Shrimp	
fresh, 4 oz.	103
cooked (fried), 4 oz.	256
canned, 4 oz.	132
Shrimp paste, 1 tbsp.	13
Shrimp scampi, 6 in butter	265
Smelts	
canned, 4 oz.	225
cooked, 4 or 5 medium	100
Soft drinks (see beverages)	
Sole, baked, 4 oz.	90
Soup (commercial canned varieties, made with water)	
asparagus, cream, 1 cup	65
bean, 1 cup	200
bean with pork, 1 cup	168
beef broth (bouillon), 1 cup	31
beef, consommé, 1 cup	70
beef noodle, 1 cup	67
celery, cream, 1 cup	86
chicken, 1 cup	75
chicken, consommé, 1 cup	22
chicken, cream, 1 cup	94
chicken gumbo, 1 cup	55
chicken noodle, 1 cup	62
chicken with rice, 1 cup	48
chicken vegetable, 1 cup	76
clam chowder, Manhattan, 1 cup	76
clam chowder, New England, 1 cup	175
green pea, 1 cup	130

Food	*Calories*
minestrone, 1 cup	105
mushroom, cream, 1 cup	134
onion, 1 cup	45
onion, French, 1 cup	125
pepper pot, 1 cup	85
potato, cream, 1 cup	85
Scotch broth, 1 cup	75
split pea, 1 cup	146
tomato, 1 cup	88
turkey noodle, 1 cup	79
vegetable, 1 cup	65
vegetable beef, 1 cup	78
vegetable with beef broth, 1 cup	78
vegetarian vegetable, 1 cup	78
Soup (dehydrated, mixed with water)	
beef noodle, 1 cup	67
chicken noodle, 1 cup	53
chicken rice, 1 cup	48
onion, 1 cup	36
pea, green, 1 cup	123
tomato vegetable, 1 cup	65
Soursop, raw, puréed, 1 cup	146
Soybeans	
fresh, 1 cup	846
cooked, 1 cup	234
sprouted seeds, fresh, 1 cup	48
sprouted seeds, cooked, 1 cup	48
Soybean curd (tofu), 1 oz.	20
Soybean flour	
full fat, 1 cup	358
low fat, 1 cup	313
Soybean oil (see oils)	
Soy sauce (see sauces)	
Spaghetti	
dry, 4 oz.	419
cooked, firm, 1 cup	192
cooked, tender, 1 cup	155
Spaghetti & meatballs in tomato sauce & cheese,	
1 cup	332

Food	Calories
Spaghetti & meatballs in tomato sauce & cheese, canned, cooked, 1 cup	258
Spaghetti in tomato sauce and cheese	
1 cup	260
canned, 1 cup	190
Spaghetti sauce, canned, with meat, 4 oz.	109
Spanish rice, cooked, 1 cup	213
Spices	0
Spinach	
fresh, chopped, 1 cup	14
cooked (boiled), 1 cup	41
canned, chopped, drained, 1 cup	49
frozen, cooked, chopped, 1 cup	47
Spot, baked, 1 oz.	84
Squab, cooked, 4 oz.	320
Squash	
acorn, fresh, 1 squash	190
acorn, cooked, mashed, 1 cup	135
butternut, baked, mashed, 1 cup	139
crookneck & straightneck (yellow), fresh, sliced, 1 cup	26
crookneck & straightneck (yellow), boiled, mashed, 1 cup	36
Hubbard, baked, mashed, 1 cup	103
scallop, boiled, mashed, 1 cup	38
zucchini, fresh, sliced, 1 cup	22
zucchini, boiled, mashed, 1 cup	29
Squid, 1 piece	85
Starch (see cornstarch)	
Stew (see beef & vegetable stew)	
St. John's-bread (see carob flour)	
Strawberries	
fresh, 1 cup	55
fresh, 1 lb.	168
canned, water pack, unsweetened, 1 cup	53
frozen, sweetened, sliced, 1 cup	278
frozen, sweetened, whole, 1 cup	235
Stuffing, bread, ½ cup	350

Food	*Calories*
Sturgeon	
cooked, 4 oz.	180
smoked, 4 oz.	168
Succotash, frozen, cooked, 1 cup	158
Sugar	
brown, packed, 1 cup	821
brown, not packed, 1 cup	541
granulated, 1 cup	770
granulated, 1 tbsp.	46
granulated, 1 tsp.	15
granulated, 1 lump (2 cubes)	19
granulated, 1 packet	23
powdered, 1 cup	462
powdered, 1 tbsp.	31
Sunflower seeds	
hulled, 1 cup	812
hulled, 1 oz.	159
Sweetbreads (cooked)	
beef, 3 oz.	272
calf, 3 oz.	143
lamb, 3 oz.	149
Sweet potatoes	
fresh, pared, 1 lb.	116
baked in skin, 4 oz.	125
boiled in skin, 4 oz.	129
boiled in skin, mashed, 1 cup	291
candied, 4 oz.	191
canned, pieces, 1 cup	216
Swordfish	
broiled with butter, 1 piece	237
broiled with butter, 4 oz.	184
Syrups (see individual kinds)	

"T"

Tamarinds, fresh, 4 oz.	130
Tangelos, 1 medium fruit	39
Tangelo juice, 1 cup	101
Tangerines, 1 medium	39

Food	Calories
Tangerine juice, canned, unsweetened, 1 cup	106
Tapioca (see puddings)	
Taro, fresh, leaves & stems, 4 oz.	45
Tartar sauce (see sauces)	
Tea (see beverages)	
Thuringer (see sausage)	
Tilefish, baked, 4 oz.	156
Tomatoes	
fresh, 1 medium	27
fresh, ½ lb.	45
boiled, 1 cup	63
canned, 1 cup	51
canned, stewed, 1 cup	64
purée, canned, 1 cup	100
Tomato chili sauce	
1 cup	284
1 tbsp.	16
Tomato juice, canned 1 cup	46
Tomato juice cocktail, 1 cup	51
Tomato ketchup (see ketchup)	
Tomato paste	
canned, 1 cup	215
canned, 4 oz.	93
Tongue (braised)	
beef, 4 oz.	277
calf, 4 oz.	181
hog, 4 oz.	287
lamb, 4 oz.	288
sheep, 4 oz.	366
Toppings (see candy & sauces)	
Tortilla, 5", 1	60
Tripe, beef, pickled, 4 oz.	70
Trout	
rainbow, canned, 4 oz.	237
fresh, brook, 4 oz.	114
Tuna	
canned, in oil, with liquid, 4 oz.	327
canned, in oil, drained, 4 oz.	224

Food	Calories
canned, in oil, drained, 1 cup	315
canned, in water, 4 oz.	144
Tuna Salad (see salads)	
Turkey	
roasted, 4 oz.	216
roasted, chopped, 1 cup	266
roasted, white meat, 4 oz.	199
roasted, white meat, chopped, 1 cup	246
roasted, dark meat, 4 oz.	230
roasted, dark meat, chopped, 1 cup	284
canned, 1 cup	414
giblets, simmered, chopped, 1 cup	338
Turkey pot pie, 4 oz.	269
Turnips	
fresh, sliced, 1 cup	39
boiled, cubed, 1 cup	36
Turnip greens	
fresh, 1 lb.	127
cooked, 1 cup	29
Turtle, canned, 4 oz.	120

"V"

Veal	
chuck and veal for stew, braised, 4 oz.	267
chuck and veal for stew, braised, chopped, 1 cup	329
loin, braised, 4 oz.	265
breast, braised, 4 oz.	344
rib roast, braised, 4 oz.	305
round, braised, 4 oz.	245
Vegetables (see individual kinds)	
Vegetable juice cocktail, canned, 1 cup	41
Vegetables, mixed, frozen, cooked, 1 cup	116
Venison, lean, roasted	166
Vienna sausage (see sausage)	
Vinegar	
cider, 1 cup	34
cider, 1 tbsp.	2
distilled, 1 cup	29

distilled, 1 tbsp.   2
Vodka (see beverages)

"W"

Waffles
  baked, round, 7" diam.   209
  baked, 4.5" square, 1   140
  frozen, 4.5" × 3.5", 1   86
Walnuts
  black, shelled, 1 oz.   178
  black, shelled, chopped, 1 cup   785
  black, shelled, chopped, 1 tbsp.   50
  black, shelled, ground, 1 cup   502
  Persian or English, shelled, halves, 1 cup   651
  Persian or English, shelled, 1 oz.   185
  Persian or English, shelled, chopped, 1 cup   781
Water chestnuts, Chinese, raw, 4 oz.   69
Watercress (see cress)
Water ice (see ices)
Watermelon
  fresh, 1 slice (4" × 8")   111
  fresh, diced, 1 cup   42
  fresh, ½ lb.   59
Weakfish, broiled in butter or margarine, 4 oz.   236
Welsh rarebit, 1 cup   415
Wheat (see cereals, flours)
Wheat germ, 1 tbsp.   29
Wheat, parboiled (see bulgur)
Whey
  fluid, 1 cup   64
  dried, 4 oz.   396
Whiskey (see beverages)
Whitefish
  cooked, stuffed, 4 oz.   244
  smoked, 4 oz.   176
White sauce (see sauces)
Wine (see beverages)

"Y"

Yams (see sweet potatoes)
Yeast
    baker's, compressed, 1 oz.   24
    baker's, dry, 1 oz.   80
    brewer's, debittered, 1 tbsp.   23
    brewer's, debittered, 1 oz.   80
Yogurt
    plain, from skimmed milk, 1 cup   123
    plain, from whole milk, 1 cup   153
    coffee, 1 cup   200
    pineapple-orange, 1 cup   260
    raspberry, 1 cup   260
    strawberry, 1 cup   260
    vanilla, 1 cup   200
Youngberries (see blackberries)

"Z"

Zwieback
    1 piece   30
    4 oz.   480

The Fast-Food Restaurant Calorie Guide

This is the most up-to-date and complete list of foods and calories from the nation's most popular fast-food restaurants. Everything from breakfast foods to special hamburgers, from French fries to pizzas, from drinks to desserts.

	Quantity	*Description*	*Calories*
Arby's	1	Junior Roast Beef	220
	1	Roast Beef	350
	1	Super Roast Beef	620
	1	Beef & Cheese	450
	1	Ham 'N Cheese	380
	1	Swiss King	660
	1	Turkey	410
	1	Turkey Deluxe	510
	1	Club	560
Arthur	2	Fish	355
Treacher's	2	Chicken	369
	7	Shrimp	381
	1	Chips	276
	1	Krunch Pups	203
	1	Coleslaw	123
	1	Lemon Luvs	276
	1	Chowder	112
	1	Fish Sandwich	440
	1	Chicken Sandwich	413

	Quantity	Description	Calories
Baskin-	1 scoop	Vanilla Ice Cream	147
Robbins	1 scoop	Chocolate Ice Cream	165
	1 scoop	Strawberry Ice Cream	141
	1 scoop	French Vanilla Ice Cream	181
	1 scoop	Chocolate Fudge Ice Cream	178
	1 scoop	Pralines N' Cream Ice Cream	177
	1 scoop	Orange Sherbet	99
	1 scoop	Daiquiri Ice	84
Burger	1	Regular Hamburger	260
Chef	1	Cheeseburger	300
	1	Double Cheeseburger	430
	1	Big Shef	540
	1	Super Shef	600
	1	Skipper's Treat	600
	1	French Fried Potatoes	190
	1	Shake	330
	1	Mariner Platter	680
	1	Rancher Platter	640
Burger	1	Cheeseburger	305
King	1	Hamburger	252
	1	Whopper	606
	1	Whaler	486
	1	Hot Dog	291
	1	French Fries	214
	1	Vanilla Shake	332
Dairy	1	Hamburger	260
Queen	1	Cheeseburger	320
	1	Big "Brazier"	460
	1	Big "Brazier" w/cheese	550
	1	Big "Brazier w/lettuce and tomato	470
	1	Super "Brazier"/the Half Pounder	780

	Quantity	Description	Calories
	1	Hot Dog	270
	1	Hot Dog w/chili	330
	1	Hot Dog w/cheese	330
	1	Fish Sandwich	400
	1	Fish Sandwich w/cheese	440
	1	French Fries	200
	1	French Fries—Large	320
	1	Onion Rings	300
Frozen Desserts			
	1	Small Cone	110
	1	Regular Cone	230
	1	Large Cone	340
	1	Small Chocolate Dipped Cone	150
	1	Regular Chocolate Dipped Cone	300
	1	Large Chocolate Dipped Cone	450
	1	Small Chocolate Sundae	170
	1	Regular Chocolate Sundae	290
	1	Large Chocolate Sundae	400
	1	Small Chocolate Malt	340
	1	Regular Chocolate Malt	600
	1	Large Chocolate Malt	840
	1	Float	330
	1	Banana Split	540
	1	Parfait	460
	1	"Fiesta" Sundae	570
	1	Freeze	520
	1	"Mr. Misty" Freeze	500
	1	"Mr. Misty" Float	440
	1	"Dilly" Bar	240
	1	"DQ" Sandwich	140
	1	"Mr. Misty" Kiss	70
Gino's	1	Hamburger	254
	1	Cheeseburger	300

	Quantity	Description	Calories
	1	Sirloiner	441
	1	Cheese Sirloiner	532
	1	Giant	569
	1	Heroburger	647
	1	Cheese Heroburger	738
	1	Fish Sandwich	450
	1	Fish Platter	650
	1	French Fries	156
	1	Apple Pie	238
	1	Vanilla Shake	310
	1	Chocolate Shake	324
	1	Coke, medium	117
	1	Root Beer, medium	122
	1	Orange, medium	140
	1	Hot Chocolate	90
	1	Milk	160
Jack	1	Hamburger	263
in	1	Cheeseburger	310
the	1	Hamburger Deluxe	260
Box	1	Cheeseburger Deluxe	314
	1	Bonus Jack Hamburger	461
	1	Jumbo Jack Hamburger	551
	1	Jumbo Jack Hamburger w/cheese	628
	1	Regular Taco	189
	1	Super Taco	285
	1	Jack Burrito	448
	1	Moby Jack Sandwich	455
	1	Jack Steak Sandwich	428
	1	Breakfast Jack Sandwich	301
	1	French Fries	270
	1	Onion Rings	351
	1	Lemon Turnover	446
	1	Apple Turnover	411
	1	Vanilla Shake	342
	1	Chocolate Shake	365
	1	Strawberry Shake	380

	Quantity	Description	Calories
	1	Ham and Cheese Omelette	425
	1	Double Cheese Omelette	423
	1	Ranchero Style Omelette	414
	1	French Toast Breakfast	537
	1	Pancakes Breakfast	626
	1	Scrambled Eggs Breakfast	719
Kentucky Fried Chicken	1	Three Piece Dinner—Original Recipe (3 pieces chicken, mashed potatoes, gravy, coleslaw, roll)	830
	1	Three Piece Dinner—Extra Crispy (3 pieces chicken, mashed potatoes, gravy, coleslaw, roll)	950
	1	Wing	151
	1	Drum	136
	1	Keel	283
	1	Rib	241
	1	Thigh	275
	1	Chicken, 9 piece cut	1892
Long John Silver	1 piece	Fish w/batter	216
	2 pieces	Fish w/batter	431
	5 pieces	Peg Legs w/batter	514
	1 fish/ 3 peg legs	Treasure Chest	525
	6 pieces	Shrimp w/batter	269
	1	Clams w/batter	465
	1	Oysters w/batter	460
	1 3-oz. serv.	Fries	250
	4-oz. serv.	Coleslaw	133
	1	Corn On The Cob	174
	3	Hush Puppies	134
McDonald's	1	Hamburger	260
	1	Cheeseburger	306

Quantity	Description	Calories
1	Quarter Pounder	420
1	Quarter Pounder w/cheese	520
1	Big Mac	540
1	Filet-O-Fish	400
1	French Fries, regular	210
1	Egg McMuffin	350
1	Pork Sausage	185
1	English Muffin, buttered	185
1	Scrambled Eggs	160
1	Hot Cakes w/butter & syrup	470
1	Chocolate Shake	365
1	Vanilla Shake	325
1	Strawberry Shake	345
1	Apple Pie	300
1	Cherry Pie	300
1	McDonaldland Cookies	295

Pizza Hut

All based on ½ of 10" pizza.

Quantity	Description	Calories
1	Thin & Crispy/beef	490
1	Thin & Crispy/pork	520
1	Thin & Crispy/cheese	450
1	Thin & Crispy/pepperoni	430
1	Thin & Crispy/supreme	510
1	Thick & Chewy/beef	620
1	Thick & Chewy/pork	640
1	Thick & Chewy/cheese	560
1	Thick & Chewy/pepperoni	560
1	Thick & Chewy/supreme	640

Rustler Steak House

Quantity	Description	Calories
4 oz.	Rib Eye Steak	224
1	Strip Steak	337
4 oz.	Chopped Steak	263
8 oz.	Chopped Steak	526
10–12 oz.	T-Bone Steak	374
1	Trail Boss Sandwich	553

	Quantity	Description	Calories
	1	Westerner Sandwich w/2 slices cheese	604
	4 oz.	Filet Mignon	308
	1	Rustler Roll	135
	1	Steak & Crab	479
	1 pat	Butter	52
	1	Salad	7
	1 tbsp.	Bleu Cheese Dressing	80
	1 tbsp.	French Dressing	60
	1 tbsp.	Thousand Island Dressing	60
	1	Jell-O, Cherry	75
	1	Pickle	2
	1	Potato Chips	82
	1	Pudding—Chocolate	144
	1	Small Iced Tea	5
	1	Small Coca Cola	117
	1	Small Root Beer	122
	8 oz.	Milk	308
Taco	1	Taco	159
Bell	1	Tostada	206
	1	Enchirito	391
	1	Bellbeefer	243
	1	Pintos 'N Cheese	231
	1	Bean Burrito	345
	1	Beefy Tostada	232
	1	Burrito Supreme	387
Wendy's	1	Single	470*
	1	Double	670*
	1	Triple	850*
	1	Single w/cheese	580*
	1	Double w/cheese	800*
	1	Triple w/cheese	1040*
	1	Chili—single	230
	1	French Fries	330
	1	Frosty Dairy Dessert	390

* lettuce, tomato, onion, pickle, mustard, ketchup included

White	1	Hamburger	164
Castle	1	Hamburger w/onion	
		& pickle	165
	2.7 oz.	French Fries	219
	1	Cheeseburger	198
	1	Fish Sandwich	200
	1	Shake	213
	3.3 oz.	Onion Rings	341

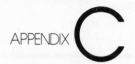

The Frozen Convenience Foods Calorie Guide

A first! This is the consummate list of *everything* in frozen foods. You will now have the calorie values for dozens of frozen dinners, entrées, pizzas, fancy vegetables, potato products . . . everything about those easy-to-prepare foods.

Banquet Dinners

Man-Pleaser Dinners	*Serving Weight*	*Calories*
Chicken	17 oz.	1016
Turkey	19 oz.	620
Meat Loaf	19 oz.	916
Salisbury Steak	19 oz.	873

Entrées	*Serving Weight*	*Calories*
Spaghetti w/Meat Sauce	8 oz.	311
Macaroni & Cheese	8 oz.	279

Meat Pies	*Serving Weight*	*Calories*
Beef	8 oz.	409
Turkey	8 oz.	415
Chicken	8 oz.	427
Tuna	8 oz.	434

Dinners	Serving Weight	Calories
Beef Chop Suey	12 oz.	282
Beef	11 oz.	312
Spaghetti & Meatballs	11.5 oz.	450
Ocean Perch	8.8 oz.	434
Haddock	8.8 oz.	419
Macaroni & Beef	12 oz.	394
Chopped Beef	11 oz.	443
Chicken & Noodles	12 oz.	374
Mexican Style	16 oz.	608
Turkey	11 oz.	293
Meat Loaf	11 oz.	412
Macaroni & Cheese	12 oz.	326
Salisbury Steak	11 oz.	390
Corned Beef Hash	10 oz.	372
Veal Parmagiana	11 oz.	421
Fried Chicken	11 oz.	530
Chicken Chow Mein	12 oz.	282
Cheese Enchilada	12 oz.	459
Italian Style	11 oz.	446
Beef Enchilada	12 oz.	479
Beans & Franks	10.8 oz.	591
Ham	10 oz.	369
Mexican Style Combination	12 oz.	571
Fish	8 oz.	382
Chicken & Dumplings	12 oz.	282
Western	11 oz.	417

Buffet Supper Products	Serving Weight	Calories
Veal Parmigiana w/Tomato Sauce	32 oz.	1563
Gravy & Salisbury Steak	32 oz.	1454
Macaroni & Beef	32 oz.	1000
Chicken & Noodles	32 oz.	764
Spaghetti & Meatballs	32 oz.	1127
Chicken & Dumplings	32 oz.	1209
Giblet Gravy & Turkey	32 oz.	564
Beef Stew	32 oz.	700

	Serving Size	Calories
Chicken Chow Mein	32 oz.	345
Gravy & Sliced Beef	32 oz.	782
Noodles & Beef	32 oz.	754
Beef Chop Suey	32 oz.	418
Beef Enchilada with Cheese & Chili Gravy	32 oz.	1118
Meat Loaf	32 oz.	1445
Macaroni & Cheese	32 oz.	1027

Cookin' Bag Products	Serving Weight	Calories
Gravy & Sliced Beef	5 oz.	116
Giblet Gravy & Sliced Turkey	5 oz.	98
Sloppy Joe	5 oz.	199
Chicken à la King	5 oz.	138
Salisbury Steak & Gravy	5 oz.	246
Creamed Chipped Beef	5 oz.	124
2 Beef Enchiladas & Sauce	6 oz.	207
B.B.Q. Sauce w/Sliced Beef	5 oz.	126
Macaroni & Cheese	8 oz.	261
Chicken Chow Mein	7 oz.	89
Beef Chop Suey	7 oz.	73
Meat Loaf	5 oz.	224
Veal Parmigiana	5 oz.	287

Birds Eye Vegetables & Potato Products

Frozen Vegetables	Serving Weight	Calories
Artichoke Hearts	3 oz.	20
Cut Asparagus	3.3 oz.	25
Asparagus Spears	3.3 oz.	25
Jumbo Asparagus Spears	3.3 oz.	25
Baby Butter Beans	3.3 oz.	140
Cut Green Beans	3 oz.	25
French Style Green Beans	3 oz.	30
Italian Green Beans	3 oz.	30
Whole Green Beans	3 oz.	25

	Serving Weight	Calories
Baby Lima Beans	3.3 oz.	120
Fordhook Lima Beans	3.3 oz.	100
Tiny Lima Beans	3.3 oz.	120
Cut Wax Beans	3 oz.	30
Baby Broccoli Spears	3.3 oz.	25
Broccoli Spears	3.3 oz.	25
Chopped Broccoli	3.3 oz.	25
Baby Brussels Sprouts	3.3 oz.	35
Brussels Sprouts	3.3 oz.	30
Cauliflower	3.3 oz.	25
Chopped Collard Greens	3.3 oz.	25
Corn on the Cob	1 ear	130
Little Ears Cob Corn	2 ears	140
Sweet Whole Kernel Corn	3.3 oz.	70
Chopped Kale	3.3 oz.	25
Mixed Vegetables	3.3 oz.	60
Chopped Mustard Greens	3.3 oz.	20
Cut Okra	3.3 oz.	25
Whole Okra	3.3 oz.	30
Chopped Onions	3 oz.	24
Small Whole Onions	4 oz.	40
Black-Eye Peas	3.3 oz.	130
Sweet Green Peas	3.3 oz.	70
Tender Tiny Peas	3.3 oz.	60
Peas & Carrots	3.3 oz.	50
Chopped Spinach	3.3 oz.	20
Leaf Spinach	3.3 oz.	20
Cooked Squash	4 oz.	50
Sliced Summer Squash	3.3 oz.	18
Zucchini Squash	3.3 oz.	16
Succotash	3.3 oz.	80
Chopped Turnip Greens	3.3 oz.	20

Combination Vegetables	Serving Weight	Calories
French Green Beans w/Mushrooms	3 oz.	30
French Green Beans w/Almonds	3 oz.	50
Broccoli w/Cheese Sauce	3.3 oz.	110

	Serving Weight	Calories
Broccoli Spears w/Hollandaise Sauce	3.3 oz.	100
Carrots w/Brown Sugar Glaze	3.3 oz.	80
Cauliflower w/Cheese Sauce	3.3 oz.	110
Green Beans & Pearl Onions	3 oz.	35
Mixed Vegetables w/Onion Sauce	2.6 oz.	110
Small Onions w/Cream Sauce	3 oz.	100
Green Peas & Cauliflower w/Cream Sauce	3.3 oz.	120
Green Peas & Pearl Onions	3.3 oz.	60
Green Peas & Potatoes w/Cream Sauce	2.6 oz.	140
Green Peas w/Cream Sauce	2.6 oz.	130
Green Peas w/Sliced Mushrooms	3.3 oz.	70
Rice & Peas w/Mushrooms	2.3 oz.	100
Creamed Spinach	3 oz.	60
Corn Jubilee	3 3 oz.	120

International Vegetables	Serving Weight	Calories
Bavarian Style Beans & Spaetzle	3.3 oz.	70
Chinese Style	3.3 oz.	20
Danish Style	3.3 oz.	30
Hawaiian Style w/Pineapple	3.3 oz.	40
Italian Style	3.3 oz.	45
Japanese Style	3.3 oz.	45
Parisian Style	3.3 oz.	30

Stir-Fry Vegetables	Serving Weight	Calories
Chinese Style	3.3 oz.	30
Japanese Style	3.3 oz.	30
Cantonese Style	3.3 oz.	50
Mandarin Style	3.3 oz.	25

Americana Vegetables	Serving Weight	Calories
New England Style	3.3 oz.	70
New Orleans Creole Style	3.3 oz.	70

	Serving Weight	Calories
Pennsylvania Dutch Style	3.3 oz.	45
San Francisco	3.3 oz.	50
Wisconsin Country Style	3.3 oz.	45

Frozen Potato Products	Serving Weight	Calories
Cottage Fries	2.8 oz.	120
Crinkle Cuts	3 oz.	110
French Fries	3 oz.	110
Hash Browns	4 oz.	70
Hash Browns O'Brien	4 oz.	60
Shredded Hash Browns	3 oz.	60
Shoestrings	3.3 oz.	140
Steak Fries	3 oz.	110
Tasti Fries, French Fries	2.5 oz.	140
Tasti Puffs, Potato Puffs	2.5 oz.	190
Tiny Taters, Potato Bites	3.2 oz.	200
Whole Peeled Potatoes	3.2 oz.	60

Buitoni Frozen Foods

Frozen Entrées	Serving Weight	Calories
Lasagna w/Meat Sauce	4 oz.	168
Meat Ravioli	4 oz.	340
Cheese Ravioli	4 oz.	316
Round Cheese Ravioli	4 oz.	272
Cheese Ravioli Parmigiana	4 oz.	152
Meat Ravioli Parmigiana	4 oz.	192
Manicotti w/o Sauce	4 oz.	196
Manicotti w/Sauce	4 oz.	176
Baked Ziti in Sauce	4 oz.	136
Shells in Sauce	4 oz.	136
Eggplant Parmigiana	4 oz.	208
Instant Cheese Pizza	4 oz.	276
Open Face Pizza	4 oz.	256

	Weight Serving	Calories
Shrimp Marinara w/Shells	4 oz.	106
Veal Parmigiana w/Spaghetti Twists	4 oz.	160
Sausage & Peppers	4 oz.	164

Celentano Italian Foods

Entrées	Serving Weight	Calories
Eggplant Parmigiana	6.5 oz.	320
Stuffed Shells (Conconi Stufati)	4.5 oz.	223
Cavatelli (Ricotta)	5 oz.	430
Manicotti	3.6 oz.	190
Lasagna	6.5 oz.	290
Ravioli (Cheese)	6.5 oz.	410

Pizza	Serving Weight	Calories
Pizza	3.7 oz.	229
Pizza Elegante	3.8 oz.	240

Celeste Pizza Products

Pizza	Serving Weight	Calories
Sausage Pizza	5.5 oz.	380
Pepperoni Pizza	5 oz.	360
Deluxe Pizza	5.9 oz.	370
Cheese Pizza	4.8 oz.	320
Sausage & Mushroom Pizza	6 oz.	380
Cheese & Mushroom Pizza	5.4 oz.	300
Sausage Pizza	4 oz.	280
Pepperoni Pizza	3.6 oz.	270
Deluxe Pizza	4.5 oz.	300
Cheese Pizza	3.5 oz.	240
Sausage & Mushroom Pizza	4.5 oz.	290
Cheese & Mushroom Pizza	4 oz.	230
Cheese Pizza Sicilian Style	5 oz.	350

Green Giant Frozen Vegetables & Entrées

Boil-in-Bag Vegetables	Serving Size	Calories
Asparagus: Cut Spears/Butter Sauce	1 cup	90
Green Beans: Cut, French Style in Butter Sauce	1 cup	70
Green Beans: Onions, Flavored w/Bacon Bits	1 cup	80
Baby Lima Beans in Butter Sauce	1 cup	220
Broccoli Spears in Butter Sauce	1 cup	90
Broccoli Cut Spears in Cheese Sauce	1 cup	130
Broccoli, Cauliflower & Carrots in Cheese Sauce	1 cup	140
Brussels Sprouts in Butter Sauce	1 cup	110
Brussels Sprouts Halves in Cheese Sauce	1 cup	170
Carrot Nuggets in Butter Sauce	1 cup	100
Cauliflower in Cheese Sauce	1 cup	130
Niblets Golden Corn, in Butter Sauce	1 cup	190
Mexican Golden Corn/Peppers in Butter Sauce	1 cup	190
Golden Corn, Cream Style	1 cup	180
White Corn Whole Kernel in Butter Sauce	1 cup	190
Mixed Vegetables in Butter Sauce	1 cup	130
Onions in Creamy Cheese Flavor Sauce	1 cup	140
Le Sueur Early Peas in Butter Sauce	1 cup	150
Sweet Peas in Butter Sauce	1 cup	150
Le Sueur Tiny Peas, Onions, Carrots in Butter Sauce	1 cup	160
Le Seur Tiny Peas, Pea Pods, & Water Chestnuts in Sauce	1 cup	180
Spinach in Butter Sauce	1 cup	90
Spinach, Creamed	1 cup	190

Boil-in-Bag Southern Recipe Vegetables	Serving Size	Calories
Black-Eyed Peas	1 cup	280
Hopping John	1 cup	300

	Weight Serving	Calories
Okra Gumbo	1 cup	220
Speckled Butter Beans	1 cup	280
Glazed Sweet Potatoes	1 cup	340
Summer Squash in Cheese Sauce	1 cup	120

Boil-in-Bag Oriental Style Combination Vegetables	Serving Size	Calories
Chinese Style Vegetables	1 cup	130
Hawaiian Style Vegetables	1 cup	200
Japanese Style Vegetables	1 cup	130

Boil-in-Bag Potato Products	Serving Size	Calories
Shoestring Potatoes in Butter Sauce	1 cup	310
Potato Slices in Butter Sauce	1 cup	210
Diced Potatoes in Sour Cream Sauce	1 cup	270
Potatoes & Sweet Peas in Bacon Cream Sauce	1 cup	240

Boil-in-Bag Toast Toppers	Serving Weight	Calories
Gravy & Sliced Beef	5 oz.	130
Gravy & Sliced Turkey	5 oz.	100
Chicken À La King	5 oz.	170
Sloppy Joe Seasoned w/Tomato Sauce & Beef	5 oz.	160
Creamed Tuna w/Peas	5 oz.	140
Welsh Rarebit Seasoned w/Cheddar & Swiss Cheese	5 oz.	220

Boil-in-Bag Entrées	Serving Weight	Calories
Macaroni & Cheese	9 oz.	330
Macaroni & Beef w/Tomato Sauce	9 oz.	240
Salisbury Steaks w/Tomato Sauce	9 oz.	390
Chicken & Noodles	9 oz.	250
Lasagna w/Meat Sauce	9 oz.	310
Beef Stew	9 oz.	160

	Weight Serving	Calories
Spaghetti & Meatballs w/Tomato Sauce	9 oz.	280
Chicken Chow Mein w/o Noodles	9 oz.	130

Boil-in-Bag Rice Originals	Serving Size	Calories
Continental—Rice w/Green Beans & Almonds	1 cup	230
Medley—Rice w/Sweet Peas & Mushrooms	1 cup	200
Pilaf—Rice w/Mushrooms & Onions	1 cup	230
White & Wild Rice	1 cup	220
White & Wild Oriental Rice w/Bean Sprouts, Pea Pods & Water Chestnuts	1 cup	230
White & Wild Medley—Rice w/Peas, Celery, Mushrooms & Almonds	1 cup	320
Rice 'N Broccoli in Cheese Sauce	1 cup	250
Verdi—Rice w/Bell Peppers & Parsley	1 cup	270

Bake & Serve Vegetables	Serving Size	Calories
Cut Broccoli in Cheese Sauce	1 cup	260
Cauliflower in Cheese Sauce	1 cup	220
Creamed Peas w/Bread Crumb Topping	1 cup	300
Spinach Soufflé	1 cup	300
Potatoes Au Gratin	1 cup	390
Potatoes Vermicelli w/Mushrooms & Cheese Sauce	1 cup	390

Oven Bake Entrées	Serving Weight	Calories
Stuffed Potatoes w/Cheese Flavored Topping	5 oz.	240
Stuffed Potatoes w/Sour Cream & Chives	5 oz.	230
Macaroni & Cheese	8 oz.	290

	Weight Serving	Calories
Salisbury Steak w/Gravy	7 oz.	290
Stuffed Green Peppers w/Beef in Creole Sauce	7 oz.	200
Stuffed Cabbage Rolls w/Beef in Tomato Sauce	7 oz.	220
Lasagna w/Meat & Sauce	7 oz.	300
Breaded Veal Parmigiana made w/Veal Patties	7 oz.	310
Chicken & Biscuits	7 oz.	200
Beef Stew & Biscuits	7 oz.	190

Poly Bag Vegetables	Serving Size	Calories
Baby Lima Beans	1 cup	150
Cut Broccoli	1 cup	30
Brussels Sprouts	1 cup	50
Cauliflower	1 cup	25
Golden Corn, Whole Kernel	1 cup	130
White Corn, Whole Kernel	1 cup	130
Small Early Peas	1 cup	100
Sweet Peas	1 cup	100
Mixed Vegetables (corn, peas, carrots, green beans, & lima beans)	1 cup	90

Jeno's Pizza Products

Pizza	Serving Weight	Calories
Cheese	6.5 oz.	420
Sausage	6.8 oz.	450
Pepperoni	6.5 oz.	450
Hamburger	6.8 oz.	440

Pizza Rolls	Serving Weight	Calories
Sausage & Cheese	3 oz.	260
Pepperoni & Cheese	3 oz.	260

	Weight Serving	Calories
Cheeseburger	3 oz.	270
Shrimp & Cheese	3 oz.	220

La Choy Frozen Products

Dinners	Serving Weight	Calories
Beef	11 oz.	342
Chicken	11 oz.	354
Pepper Oriental	11 oz.	349
Shrimp	11 oz.	325

Entrées	Serving Weight	Calories
Beef Chow Mein	16 oz.	97
Chicken Chow Mein	16 oz.	108
Fried Rice & Pork	12 oz.	216
Pepper Oriental	15 oz.	110
Shrimp Chow Mein	16 oz.	73
Sweet & Sour Pork	15 oz.	245

Egg Rolls	Serving Weight	Calories
Chicken	6.5 oz.	120
Lobster	6.5 oz.	108
Meat & Shrimp	6.5 oz.	108
Meat & Shrimp	7.5 oz.	102
Shrimp	6.5 oz.	104

La Pizzeria Pizza

Pizza	Serving Weight	Calories
Combination	6.8 oz.	420
	6.1 oz.	380
Sausage	6.5 oz.	430
	5.8 oz.	380
Pepperoni	5.3 oz.	330

	Weight Serving	Calories
Cheese	5 oz.	290
Thick Crust Cheese	6.2 oz.	410

Morton Frozen Dinners

Frozen Dinners	Serving Weight	Calories
Beans & Franks	10.8 oz.	530
Beef	10 oz.	290
Boneless Chicken	10 oz.	230
Chicken Croquette	10.3 oz.	410
Chicken 'N Dumpling	11 oz.	300
Chicken 'N Noodles	10.3 oz.	220
Fish	8.8 oz.	265
Fried Chicken	11 oz.	460
Haddock	9 oz.	350
Ham	10 oz.	450
Italian Style	11 oz.	300
Macaroni & Beef	10 oz.	240
Macaroni & Cheese	11 oz.	350
Meat Loaf Dinner	11 oz.	370
Meat Ravioli	10 oz.	330
Salisbury Steak	11 oz.	280
Shrimp	7.8 oz.	400
Spaghetti & Meatball	11 oz.	360
Spaghetti & Sauce	11 oz.	240
Turkey	11 oz.	370
Turkey Tetrazzini	11 oz.	470
Western Round Up	11 oz.	400
Fried Chicken	6.4 oz.	440

Country Table Dinners	Serving Weight	Calories
Chicken 'N Dumplings	15 oz.	570
Fried Chicken	15 oz.	740
Meat Loaf	15 oz.	475
Salisbury Steak	15 oz.	430

Sliced Beef	14 oz.	540
Sliced Turkey	15 oz.	600

Pies & Casseroles	*Serving Weight*	*Calories*
Beef Pot Pie	8 oz.	390
Chicken Pot Pie	8 oz.	360
Tuna Pot Pie	8 oz.	400
Turkey Pot Pie	8 oz.	400
Macaroni & Cheese Casserole	8 oz.	310
Spaghetti & Meat Casserole	8 oz.	250

Mrs. Paul's Fish & Vegetable Products

Fish Products	*Serving Weight*	*Calories*
Deviled Crabs	3 oz.	160
Deviled Crab Miniatures	3.5 oz.	220
Fried Scallops	3.5 oz.	210
Fried Fish Fillets	4 oz.	220
Fried Haddock Fillets	4 oz.	230
Fried Flounder Fillets	4 oz.	220
Fried Ocean Perch Fillets	4 oz.	250
Buttered Fish Fillets	5 oz.	310
Fish Cakes	4 oz.	210
Beach Haven Fish Cakes	4 oz.	220
Clam Sticks	4 oz.	240
Fried Clams	2.5 oz.	270
Deviled Clams	3 oz.	180
Fried Shrimp	3 oz.	170
Shrimp Sticks	3.2 oz.	190
Shrimp Cakes	3 oz.	150
Fish Sticks	3 oz.	150
Fish Parmesan	5 oz.	220
Fish Au Gratin	5 oz.	250
Light Batter Fish Sticks	3.5 oz.	230
Light Batter Scallops	3.5 oz.	200

Sole w/Lemon Butter	4.5 oz.	160
Flounder w/Lemon Butter	4.5 oz.	150
Scallops w/Butter & Cheese	7 oz.	260
Supreme Light Batter Fish Fillets	3.3 oz.	220
Crab Crepes	5.5 oz.	240
Shrimp Crepes	5.5 oz.	250
Clam Crepes	5.5 oz.	280
Scallop Crepes	5.5 oz.	220

	Serving	
Frozen Vegetables	*Weight*	*Calories*
Candied Sweet Potatoes—Orange	4 oz.	180
Candied Sweet Potatoes—Yellow	4 oz.	180
Candied Sweets 'N Apples	4 oz.	160
Fried Onion Rings	2.5 oz.	150
Fried Eggplant Sticks	3.5 oz.	260
Fried Eggplant Slices	3 oz.	230
Eggplant Parmesan	5.5 oz.	250
Light Batter Zucchini Sticks	3 oz.	180
Corn Fritters	4 oz.	260
Apple Fritters	4 oz.	240
Light Batter Broccoli & Cheese	2.5 oz.	150
Light Batter Cauliflower & Cheese	2.6 oz.	120

Ore-Ida Potato & Vegetable Products

	Serving	
Potato Products	*Weight*	*Calories*
Golden Crinkles	3 oz.	130
Golden Fries	3 oz.	130
Shoe-Strings	3 oz.	170
Pixie Crinkles	3 oz.	170
Country Style Dinner Fries	3 oz.	120
Cottage Fries	3 oz.	140
Crispers	3 oz.	230
Heinz Self Sizzling Fries	3 oz.	160
Heinz Self Sizzling Crinkles	3 oz.	160
Heinz Self Sizzling Shoestrings	3 oz.	220

Southern Style Hash Browns	3 oz.	70
Shredded Hash Browns	6 oz.	120
Tater Tots Plain	3 oz.	160
Tater Tots w/Onions	3 oz.	160
Tater Tots w/Bacon Flavor	3 oz.	150
Small Whole Peeled Potatoes	3 oz.	70
O'Brien Potatoes	3 oz.	60
Potatoes w/Butter Sauce	3 oz.	120
Potatoes w/Butter Sauce & Onions	3 oz.	130

	Serving	
Vegetables	*Weight*	*Calories*
Stew Vegetables	3 oz.	60
Onion Ringers	2 oz.	160
Chopped Onions	2 oz.	20
Whole Kernel Corn	3 oz.	100
Cob Corn	4.5 oz.	140

Ronzoni Italian Foods

	Serving	
Frozen Entrées	*Weight*	*Calories*
Lasagne (w/Ricotta Cheese)	4 oz.	140
Linguine (w/white clam sauce)	4 oz.	120
Fettuccine Alfredo	4 oz.	190
Baked Ziti	4 oz.	115

Stokely-Van Camp Vegetables & Fruit

	Serving	
Vegetables	*Weight*	*Calories*
Asparagus, Cut	4 oz.	35
Asparagus Spears	4 oz.	30
Beans, Baby Butter	3.3 oz.	140
Beans, Baby Green Lima	3.3 oz.	120
Beans, Fordhook Lima	3.3 oz.	100
Beans, Green, Cut	3 oz.	30
Beans, Green, French Cut	3.3 oz.	30
Broccoli, Chopped	3.3 oz.	25
Broccoli, Cut	3 oz.	25

Broccoli, Spears	3.3 oz.	30
Brussels Sprouts	3.3 oz.	40
Carrots, Cut	3 oz.	35
Cauliflower	3.3 oz.	25
Corn	3.3 oz.	90
Corn, Cream Style	3.3 oz.	90
Peas	3.3 oz.	70
Peas & Carrots	3.3 oz.	50
Potatoes, Crinkle Cut	3 oz.	120
Spinach, Chopped	3.3 oz.	25
Spinach, Leaf	3.3 oz.	25
Squash	3 oz.	30
Succotash	3.3 oz.	100
Vegetables, Mixed	3.3 oz.	60
Vegetables, Stew	4 oz.	60
Broccoli Florentine	3.3 oz.	30
Chuckwagon Corn	3.3 oz.	90
Vegetables Del Sol	3 oz.	25
Vegetables Milano	3 oz.	45
Vegetables Orient	3 oz.	25
Vegetables Rio	3 oz.	35
Vegetables Romano	3 oz.	40

Fruit	Serving Weight	Calories
Red Raspberries	5 oz.	160
Strawberry Halves	5 oz.	160
Whole Strawberries	4 oz.	110

Stouffer Frozen Foods

Entrées	Serving Weight	Calories
Macaroni & Beef w/Tomatoes	5.8 oz.	190
Macaroni & Cheese	6 oz.	260
Creamed Chicken	6.5 oz.	300
Tuna Noodle Casserole	5.8 oz.	200
Stuffed Peppers	7.8 oz.	225

Creamed Chipped Beef	5.5 oz.	235
Lasagna	10.5 oz.	385
Beef Stroganoff	9.8 oz.	390
Salisbury Steak	6 oz.	250
Beef Stew	10 oz.	310
Spinach Soufflé	4 oz.	135
Chicken À La King	9.5 oz.	330
Green Pepper Steak	10.5 oz.	350
Potatoes Au Gratin	3.8 oz.	135
Scalloped Potatoes	4 oz.	126
Turkey Tet	6 oz.	240
Corn Soufflé	4 oz.	155
Broccoli Au Gratin	5 oz.	170
Escalloped Chicken	5.8 oz.	250
Chicken Divan	8.5 oz.	335
Noodles Romanoff	4 oz.	170
Spaghetti	14 oz.	445
Shrimp & Scallops Mariner	10.2 oz.	400
Ribs of Beef	5.8 oz.	350
Swedish Meatballs	11 oz.	475
Teriyaki	10 oz.	365
Chicken Cacciatore	11.2 oz.	310
Chicken Paprikash	10.5 oz.	385
Beef Hash	5.8 oz.	265

	Serving Weight	*Calories*
Pizza		
Cheese	5.2 oz.	330
Deluxe	6.3 oz.	400
Pepperoni	5.6 oz.	400
Sausage	6 oz.	420

	Serving Weight	*Calories*
Meat Pies		
Chicken	10 oz.	500
Beef	10 oz.	550
Turkey	10 oz.	460

Swanson Dinners & Entrées

Frozen TV Dinners	Complete Dinner Serving Weight	Calories
Barbecue Flavored Fried Chicken	11.3 oz.	530
Beans & Beef Patties	11 oz.	500
Beans & Franks	11.3 oz.	550
Beef	11.5 oz.	370
Beef Enchiladas	15 oz.	570
Chopped Sirloin Beef	10 oz.	460
Crispy Fried Chicken	10.8 oz.	650
Fish 'N Chips	10.3 oz.	450
Fried Chicken	11.5 oz.	570
German Style	11.8 oz.	430
Ham	10.3 oz.	380
Italian Style	13 oz.	420
Loin of Pork	11.3 oz.	470
Macaroni & Beef	12 oz.	400
Macaroni & Cheese	12.5 oz.	390
Meat Loaf	10.8 oz.	530
Meatballs	11.8 oz.	400
Mexican Style Combination	16 oz.	600
Noodles & Chicken	10.3 oz.	390
Polynesian Style	13 oz.	490
Salisbury Steak	11.5 oz.	500
Spaghetti & Meatballs	12.5 oz.	410
Swiss Steak	10 oz.	350
Turkey	11.5 oz.	360
Veal Parmigiana	12.3 oz.	520
Western Style	11.8 oz.	460

Three Course Dinners	Complete Dinner Serving Weight	Calories
Beef	15 oz.	490
Fried Chicken	15 oz.	630

	Complete Dinner Serving Weight	Calories
Salisbury Steak	16 oz.	490
Turkey	16 oz.	520

Hungry-Man Dinners	Complete Dinner Serving Weight	Calories
Hungry-Man Barbecue Fried Chicken	16.5 oz.	760
Hungry-Man Boneless Chicken	19 oz.	730
Hungry-Man Chopped Beef Steak	18 oz.	730
Hungry-Man Fish 'n Chips	15.8 oz.	760
Hungry-Man Fried Chicken	15.8 oz.	910
Hungry-Man Lasagna w/Meat	17.8 oz.	740
Hungry-Man Salisbury Steak	17 oz.	870
Hungry-Man Sliced Beef	17 oz.	540
Hungry-Man Spaghetti & Meatballs	18.5 oz.	660
Hungry-Man Turkey	19 oz.	740
Hungry-Man Veal Parmigiana	20.5 oz.	910
Hungry-Man Western Style	17.8 oz.	890

Frozen TV Entrées	Complete Entrée Serving Weight	Calories
Chicken Nibbles w/French Fries	6 oz.	370
Fish 'N Chips	5 oz.	290
French Toast w/Sausages	4.5 oz.	300
Fried Chicken w/Whipped Potatoes	7 oz.	360
Gravy & Sliced Beef w/Whipped Potatoes	8 oz.	190
Meatballs w/Gravy & Whipped Potatoes	9.3 oz.	330
Meatloaf w/Tomato Sauce & Whipped Potatoes	9 oz.	330
Pancakes & Sausage	6 oz.	500

	Complete Entrée Serving Weight	Calories
Salisbury Steak w/Crinkle Potatoes	5.5 oz.	370
Scrambled Eggs & Sausage w/Coffee Cake	6.3 oz.	460
Spaghetti in Tomato Sauce w/Breaded Veal	8.3 oz.	290
Turkey-Gravy-Dressing & Chipped Potatoes	8.8 oz.	260

Frozen Meat Pies	Complete Pie Serving Weight	Calories
Beef	8 oz.	430
Chicken	8 oz.	450
Turkey	8 oz.	450
Macaroni & Cheese	7 oz.	230

Hungry-Man Meat Pies	Complete Pie Serving Weight	Calories
Hungry-Man Beef	16 oz.	770
Hungry-Man Chicken	16 oz.	780
Hungry-Man Sirloin Burger	16 oz.	800
Hungry-Man Turkey	16 oz.	790

Hungry-Man Entrées	Complete Entrée Serving Weight	Calories
Hungry-Man Barbecue Chicken	12 oz.	550
Hungry-Man Fried Chicken	12 oz.	620
Hungry-Man Lasagna	12.8 oz.	540
Hungry-Man Salisbury Steak	12.5 oz.	640
Hungry-Man Sliced Beef	12.3 oz.	330
Hungry-Man Turkey	13.3 oz.	380

Taste O'Sea Frozen Fish Products

Cod Fish	Serving Weight	Calories
Raw Breaded Cod Portions	4 oz.	130
Breaded "Banquet Style" Cod Portions	4 oz.	140
Golden Fried Moby Dicks	5.2 oz.	310
Golden Fried Skinless Cod Sticks	4 oz.	260
Golden Fried Cod Portions Long	4 oz.	190
Batter Dipt Cod Wedgies (Oven Bake)	3 oz.	210
Batter Fried Cod Wedgies	3 oz.	170

Pollock Fish	Serving Weight	Calories
Breaded Pollock Squares	4 oz.	130
Golden Fried Pollock Portions Long	3 oz.	160
Golden Fried Fish Sticks	4 oz.	180
Batter Dipt Pollock Wedgies	3 oz.	200
Batter Fried Pollock Wedgies	3 oz.	150

Whiting Fish	Serving Weight	Calories
Golden Fried Whiting	3.6 oz.	180
Batter Dipt Whiting	3 oz.	210
Batter Fried Whiting Wedgies	3 oz.	140

Van de Kamp's Frozen Meals

Entrées	Serving Weight	Calories
Fish Sticks	5 oz.	310
French Fried Halibut	4 oz.	270
French Fried Fish Fillets	6 oz.	440
Tartar Sauce Packet	1 oz.	160
French Fried Fish & Chips	8 oz.	500
French Fried Fish Kabobs	4 oz.	260
Seafood Sauce Packet	1 oz.	25
Fillet of Fish w/Potatoes in Cheese Sauce	11.5 oz.	380

	Serving Weight	Calories
Fillet of Fish w/Seasoned Rice	11.5 oz.	470
Macaroni & Cheese	5 oz.	150
Chicken Stuffed Pie	7.5 oz.	480
Chicken Gravy Cup	3 oz.	50
Chicken Pie	7.5 oz.	520
Cheese Enchilada	7.5 oz.	330
Beef Enchilada	7.5 oz.	270
4 Cheese Enchiladas	9.5 oz.	400
4 Beef Enchiladas	9.5 oz.	370
Combination Pizza	5.9 oz.	310
Cheese Pizza	4.8 oz.	360
French Fried Haddock	4.8 oz.	330
French Fried Perch	4.8 oz.	290
Shrimp & Chips	7 oz.	350
Battered Fish Dinner	11 oz.	540
Mexican Combination Dinner	11 oz.	421

Dinners	Serving Weight	Calories
Fillet of Fish Dinner	12 oz.	300
Shrimp Dinner	10 oz.	370
Taquito Dinner		
Beef Enchilada Dinner	12 oz.	420
Cheese Enchilada Dinner	12 oz.	430
Mexican Style Dinner	12 oz.	480

Weaver Frozen Poultry Products

Batter Dipped Chicken	Serving Weight	Calories
Thighs & Drumsticks	4 oz.	306
Breast Pieces	4 oz.	304
Party Pack	4 oz.	344

Dutch Frye Chicken	Serving Weight	Calories
Regular	4 oz.	323
Thighs & Drumsticks	4 oz.	326

	Serving Weight	Calories
Breast Pieces	4 oz.	331
Party Pack	4 oz.	360
Drumsticks	4 oz.	271

Dutch Entrées	Serving Weight	Calories
Au Gratin	4 oz.	166
Croquettes	4 oz.	324

Weight Watchers Frozen Products

Casseroles	Serving Weight	Calories
Eggplant Parmigiana	13 oz.	250
Ziti Macaroni	13 oz.	370
Lasagna	13 oz.	380
Cannelloni Florentine	13 oz.	450
Turkey Tetrazzini	13 oz.	400
Sausage/Cheese/Tomato Pie	7 oz.	390
Cheese/Tomato Pie	6 oz.	380
Veal Stuffed Pepper	13 oz.	360
Chicken Creole	13 oz.	250

3-Compartment Meals	Serving Weight	Calories
Chicken Oriental Style	15 oz.	350
Chicken w/Stuffing	16 oz.	410
Flounder	16 oz.	260
Haddock	16 oz.	250
Perch	16 oz.	300
Sole	16 oz.	250
Sirloin of Beef	16 oz.	510
Sliced Breast of Turkey	16 oz.	350
Stuffed Turbot	16 oz.	420

2-Compartment Meals	Serving Weight	Calories
Sole	9.5 oz.	210
Flounder	8.5 oz.	170

	Serving Weight	Calories
Perch	8.5 oz.	210
Stuffed Haddock	8.75 oz.	170
Veal Parmigiana	9.5 oz.	230
Chicken Livers & Onions	10.5 oz.	220
Beef Steak	10 oz.	390
Turbot	8 oz.	310
Chicken (White Meat)	9 oz.	290
Chicken Parmigiana	9 oz.	190
Chicken Divan	9 oz.	250

Index